LOSE
THAT
BABY
FAT!

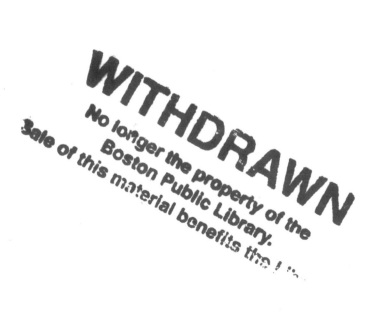

LOSE THAT BABY FAT!

Bouncing Back
the First Year
After Having a Baby

LaReine Chabut

with Foreword by Sheryl A. Ross, M.D.

M. Evans
Lanham • New York • Boulder • Toronto • Oxford

Published by M. Evans
An imprint of The Rowman & Littlefield Publishing Group, Inc.
4501 Forbes Boulevard, Suite 200, Lanham, Maryland 20706

Designed and Typeset by Chrissy Kwasnik

Library of Congress Cataloging-in-Publication Data

Chabut, LaReine.
  Lose that baby fat! : bouncing back the first year after having a baby
/ LaReine Chabut ; with foreword by Sheryl A. Ross.
     p. cm.
  Includes index.
  ISBN 1-59077-102-8; 978-1-59077-102-0
  1. Postnatal care. 2. Mothers--Health and hygiene. 3. Physical fitness for women. 4. Exercise for women. I. Title.
  RG801.C43 2006
  618.6--dc22
                           2005025099

The information contained in this book is not intended to serve as a replacement for professional medical advice. Any use of the information in this book is at the reader's discretion. The author and publisher specifically disclaim any and all liability arising directly or indirectly from the use or application of any information contained in this book. A health care professional should be consulted regarding your specific situation.

To My Daughter Bella,

Who gives me so much love every day
and inspires me to be a better mom.

I Love You,
Mommy

Contents

Acknowledgements

IT'S TOUGH TO SIT ENDLESSLY for hours on end and come up with creative thoughts when you're writing. But both my husband Bobby and my daughter Bella made me feel like I could accomplish anything. And because this book is so personal and really comes from my heart, I want to thank both of them for being there and giving me the encouragement I needed along the way.

My editor, Matt Harper, who gave me an unlimited budget (ha!) and helped me to write the best book I could, also deserves a big thanks along with my agent, Danielle Egan Miller, who found it a home at M. Evans.

Patricia Ballesteros, who coaches seeing-impaired clients, was the technical advisor for the exercises. Patty really brought her natural talent and enthusiasm as a trainer to the photo shoot. Needless to say, she has an eye for detail. Thanks so much, Patty.

Tilden Patterson is the amazing photographer who suggested we shoot at a home studio to give the photos a more natural feel. I thank him so much for that and for making me look like a hot mama along with the help of makeup artist, Kerry Herta.

NIKE and Saga Hamilton also deserve big thanks for supplying all the clothing and for being a big supporter of mine since the beginning of my career. Thanks, guys, for continuing to believe in me . . .

A special thanks to SPRI Products and Toni Eckert for supplying all of the outstanding equipment for the photo shoot and on such a tight deadline!

Molly and Allison Lorber, Tracy and Bennett Rosenthal—I thank you all for the great pictures.

And a big thanks to all the moms: Kelly Bonanno, Laura Stanley, Erin Newman, Charity Brockman, Kathleen Anne Hunt, Lara Starr, Heather McDonald Tobias, Cheryl Dorfman, Janay Schrier, Adele Clarkson, and Elana Cornelius for bravely sharing their stories and revealing their insecurities for this book. I thank you all from the bottom of my heart!

Author's Note

IN 2001 B.B. (Before Bella, my daughter), I had time to think of only me, me, and well, me. I would take whatever yoga or kickboxing class I wanted at the drop of a hat, go to the movies whenever the mood struck me or grab a bite to eat at some hip new restaurant. Then I had a baby. And as everyone was so quick to tell me when I was pregnant—my life did indeed change overnight.

Now I work out at home, rent lots of movies, and make dinner for my family instead of going out. But am I complaining? Absolutely not! I wouldn't trade my life as a busy mom for anything in the world. I really do consider it the most important thing I'll ever do in this lifetime. Now I just have to manage my time a little bit better so I can fit everything I need to do into one long day.

But would I trade my post-baby body for my pre-baby shape? Well, that's an entirely different story. And here's my question: Why didn't anyone tell me I would still look six months pregnant when I came home from the hospital after giving birth? And why did some people (I'm not going to name any names here, so don't worry) tell me to bring my jeans to the hospital because I would be able to wear them home? Ridiculous! What planet are these people from? Certainly not this one where according to the American College of Obstetricians, 80 percent of women who give birth each year gain more than the recommended 25 to 35 pounds while they're pregnant. Yes, believe it or not, after talking to my friends and many other women, I found that most of them gained more than the recommended 25 to 35 pounds. Darn! If we only knew now what we didn't know then—that it would be tough to take it all off. Especially those last 10 pounds!

And so I was inspired to write *Lose That Baby Fat!* to let you know that if any of the above sounds familiar, you are in good company—no, make that great company! My book is not geared to supermodels and actresses looking to rapidly regain their pre-pregnancy shape or to lose 30 pounds in 30 days. Rather, it is a practical guide and reality-based fitness program created just for you—the real mom trying to shed unwanted pounds the first year after having a baby. The real mom that doesn't have a personal trainer, nanny, personal chef, or timely tummy tuck!

And the greatest thing about this book is that I've broken down the entire first-year-post-baby into a simple and easy-to-follow month-by-month format. Each month I give you specific goals you can easily achieve along with a laundry list that details how you may be feeling and looking each step of the way. I call them benchmarks, just like the benchmarks you use for your baby as they grow and change throughout each stage of their life.

And last but definitely not least, I offer personal stories, anecdotes, and questions from other new moms like yourself that bravely discuss how different their bodies look and feel after giving birth (a special thanks to all the moms that shared their letters with me). So if you lose weight by following the *Lose That Baby Fat!* program, get a renewed positive self-image, and have a few laughs while you're reading this book, then I guess I've done my job—and that is to help you through this miraculous and hectic time with a newborn and an unfamiliar body. So let's get started . . . before the baby wakes up!

Foreword

WHAT YOU NEED TO KNOW BEFORE GETTING STARTED

As the mother of three active boys and a doctor with a busy practice, I know very well what you are going through as a new mom. In fact, you're probably having difficulty finding the time to read this book right now. Yes, the postpartum period tends to be an emotional roller coaster for all of us and by starting to work out immediately following the birth of your child, you stand to benefit in a number of areas. Exercise improves your metabolism, thereby giving you more energy, which helps to get rid of the extra weight gained in pregnancy and, mentally, reduces stress and improves your sense of well-being. The psychological benefit of getting into an exercise regimen is a powerful reason alone to start some form of exercise as soon as the baby is delivered.

As the medical consultant for *Expecting Fitness* and *Two at a Time: Having Twins with Jane Seymour*, I know how many concerns you may have when it comes to exercise and getting back in shape during this time. I've answered for you in the following pages the most frequently asked questions posed to me by my patients. If you find you have a question I haven't answered here, be sure to ask your OB/GYN to set your mind at ease and to help you find some comfort as you make the transition into motherhood.

WHEN YOU SHOULD BEGIN WORKING OUT

How soon you resume exercising after a vaginal delivery will vary according to your physical and mental condition, previous exercise history prior to and during pregnancy, and your delivery experience. If you had a traumatic delivery and/or had an episiotomy you may not be able to start even the easiest of exercises until three to four weeks postpartum due to the time it takes for your episiotomy sutures to heal. If you had an uncomplicated delivery with minimal trauma to your perineum, you can then start light exercise as soon as you feel up to it.

Kegel exercises (a woman can identify these pelvic floor muscles by starting and stopping her flow of urine) as given in Chapter 1 of this book should start during pregnancy and continue as an ongoing exercise for women after giving birth. Doing this passive exercise twenty to thirty times a day will promote strong pelvic floor muscles and help reduce the incidence of urinary incontinence following a vaginal delivery. A vaginal delivery will cause the weakening of these pelvic floor muscles so Kegel exercises should always be a regular part of any exercise routine. As an added bonus, Kegel exercises can enhance the sexual experience for both women and men!

Walking is another excellent exercise as discussed in Chapter 2 of this book and is perfect for this time period until you are ready to transition into a more advanced form of cardiovascular exercise. You should remember that your joints are still loose during the first six weeks postpartum, which will interfere with your coordination and balance so you want to start out slowly and with your doctor's blessing.

On the other hand, having a Cesarean section is a major surgical procedure. It takes four weeks just for the sutures to dissolve following a C-section. With this in mind, an exercise regimen can be initiated based on the same criteria as mentioned above with a vaginal delivery. Light walking, stretching exercises, and Kegels can always be incorporated but waiting to do more intense cardiovascular exercises until after your postpartum visit with your obstetrician is best.

GETTING YOUR BODY BACK

Returning to your original pre-pregnant body depends on a number of factors: your exercise regimen during pregnancy, the amount of weight you gained, your mode of delivery, and your motivation to start working out during the postpartum period. Those women that I see at six weeks postpartum who have only 10 more pounds to lose are the lucky ones and are the exceptions. I tell my patients that it took nine months to go through this process and get to this point, so you have to wait at least nine months to one year to get your original body back. Consistency, motivation, determination, and genetics are the factors toward your success.

THIS BOOK WILL HELP YOU ACHIEVE SUCCESS!

In *Lose That Baby Fat!*, you will find answers to your concerns about how you should be feeling after giving birth and learn how you can fit in exercise each month to help you establish good fitness habits now and for the future. The other aspects of this book that make it so unique and important for new moms to read also deserve a mention:

- Each chapter starts out with a list that includes *How You May Be Feeling*, and *How Your Body May Look* which makes this book invaluable for women by giving them something to identify with during this important and ever-changing time in their lives.

- The book's supportive and encouraging tone, through the use of letters from real reader moms, is very beneficial and comforting. It also helps new moms feel they are in good company when they don't have their bodies back as soon as they would like.

- The book's breakdown of the workouts that allow women to work on a different body part each month is both practical and effective. It also helps women benchmark their success by giving them specific goals each month that they can easily achieve.

There is no question that regular exercise sessions are recommended for all healthy pregnant and postpartum women because of the favorable cardiovascular, metabolic, and biomechanical effects. Realities and perceptions of exercise in pregnancy and during the postpartum period have changed dramatically over the past ten years. In LaReine Chabut's book, *Lose That Baby Fat!,* she knowledgeably, delicately, and humorously discusses ways to get back into shape in a realistic time frame. Her month-to-month program gives new moms a tangible schedule to get back their original shape in a healthy, unintimidating, and manageable fashion. This book is an excellent, well-balanced source of information that should find its way to each postpartum woman who desires to take control of her body during this emotionally and physically difficult time.

Sheryl A. Ross, M.D.

St. John's Hospital

Santa Monica, California

1

Getting Started:
No Excuses!

How Your Body May Look:
Still six months pregnant

How You May Be Feeling:
Baby blues for the first few weeks after birth

Equipment Needed:
Your own Kegel muscles, to help accelerate
the tightening of the pelvic floor, which
happens by Week 6

● ○ ○ ○ ○ ○

○ ○ ○ ○ ○ ○

CONGRATULATIONS, MOM! You've just done something spectacular: you've given birth to a new little person who is going to change your life forever. For the past nine months or so, your body has worked in truly amazing ways to nourish and grow another human being. And you've survived the most challenging part of the process: labor and delivery. You probably feel that you've been stretched, pulled, and twisted in ways you never thought possible. It really did feel like running a marathon, didn't it? But every ounce of discomfort, every moment of pain was well worth it when you hold your new baby in your arms.

WHAT YOU CAN EXPECT YOUR BODY TO LOOK AND FEEL LIKE

Now that you're back home and getting to know your new arrival, you can't help but notice how you've changed since having that baby. Your body looks very, very different, doesn't it? Whether or not you exercised throughout your pregnancy, you are likely to not only be carrying noticeable extra weight, but you're squishy in places you used to be firm, you may have extra sags or rolls of skin in places where you were once taut, and your tummy . . . well, let's just say it's still probably kind of big and looks like you have a Shar-Pei sitting on your lap. It's not pretty. And your breasts? Let's just agree that they have a mind of their own, shall we?

And then there's the fatigue. Between changing diapers, feedings every three or four hours, doing the laundry, and trying to keep the rest of your life in some semblance of order, you probably haven't had a full night's sleep in weeks. Who would've thought that you could actually function day-in, day-out, while feeling so tired? And who knew it would be so tough to leave the house, especially when you're toting a new baby around with you everywhere? And I do mean everywhere! Did you ever think for a moment that going to the bank to use the ATM machine would be so difficult? Or getting a shower would become such a luxury? I bet you didn't—and neither did I.

Just as a reality check, see if this story sounds at all familiar. You get to the bank to make a deposit, and then realize you have two choices. Choice number one is to simply leave the baby in the car since you're only ten steps away and it would be so much easier to make that deposit solo. And choice number two is to undo the baby seat carrier, take the baby and the carrier out of the car, set it on the ground, close the car door, pick it back up, make the deposit, then retrace your steps and do it all over again in reverse. Whew! I'm tired just thinking about it! My point is—and I'm sure you know what I'm talking about by now—I never really realized how daunting it would be to just get out of the house! And work out? *Are you crazy?!* It's just too much to think about.

YES, YOU CAN EXERCISE

Believe it or not, there is a way to fit exercising back into your day and a way to lose that baby weight in a safe, healthy, and timely manner. Another congratulations, Mom. If you're reading this book right now, you have taken the first step in a yearlong process that will forever change how you feel about your post-baby body and will ultimately change how you look.

This book, *Lose That Baby Fat!,* will help you, the new mom, achieve a series of realistic fitness benchmarks for the entire first year after having your baby and will help you shed those pregnancy pounds. Every month, I'll provide you with a detailed list of what you can expect your body to look and feel like—from the first six weeks after giving birth through the entire first year. The fitness program included here is tailor-made specifically for you, the busy mom who can't find time to shower, let alone work out for an hour or more each day. Month-by-post-pregnancy-month, each chapter includes 10-minute workouts highlighting a different body part. Yes, doing a 10-minute workout first thing in the morning and another 10-minute workout later in the afternoon is enough beneficial, daily exercise to jumpstart your metabolism and help you start shedding pounds. The exercises are designed so they can be varied in intensity and duration as you gain (or regain) strength, flexibility, and endurance during those first twelve months after your little bundle of joy arrives.

Quite often throughout *Lose That Baby Fat!,* I make mention of the "healthy way" to do things. By that I mean the best way for you to accomplish your goals and feel good about yourself, one day at a time, so that eventually you will get to where you want to be. No crash dieting, no unrealistic workouts that won't fit into your schedule, and no suffering to be thin—only practical and rewarding things you can learn from other new moms and do for yourself today.

NO MORE EXCUSES!

When that new baby arrives, you can find an excuse to get out of pretty much anything—including exercise. Below are some common complaints about exercise from moms just like you. These common excuses will shed a little light on the reasons why many moms put off exercise and on how to avoid falling into those traps.

" I'm too tired from changing poopy diapers. "

"I'm just too tired and can't find the time with all these diaper changes. Who knew a tiny baby could poop so much! Will exercising really give me a boost of energy?"

Yes! Exercise will actually help decrease the fatigue from not sleeping as well as increase your energy level by speeding up your circulation and jumpstarting your metabolism. The walking program that I offer for the first twelve weeks post-pregnancy will help you conquer that feeling of tiredness and revitalize your mood along with your body. As you progress through my program into your third month post pregnancy, I offer a series of practical exercises that will help you gain strength and redefine your tummy area with a series of abdominal strengtheners so you can tone and tighten the areas that were stretched out during pregnancy.

" I'm breast-feeding. "

> "I'm breast-feeding and I am hungry all the time. I can't seem to stop eating. I feel like the baby is sucking everything right out of me. Plus, everybody has told me I can eat whatever I want because I'll burn the calories and my baby weight right off! Is this true?"

Tough question (and probably the biggest misconception when it comes to losing weight after having a baby) so I'm going to provide you with a detailed explanation to dispel the myth once and for all about breast-feeding and losing weight!

Although breast-feeding actually can cause weight loss for a nursing mommy, it expends just 500 extra calories a day (which is an apple, a slice of cheese, and a yogurt). This is where the dilemma comes in! Because most women who breast-feed have a larger than normal appetite (as described in the letter), you will not be able to lose any weight and regain your pre-pregnancy shape if you take in more calories than you burn. So, although breast-feeding can actually cause weight loss, for a breast-feeding mommy it is more a matter of *gradual* weight loss through moderate exercise because you cannot safely diet as soon as a non-breast-feeding mommy can. I am a big supporter of breast-feeding (good for baby, good for mommy) so I have designed a program that will help you keep up your energy—which is already low from all of the responsibilities of caring for a new baby—and will help you seek gradual weight loss that is prescribed for breast-feeding moms, which is no more than 2 ½ pounds a month. This pace will allow you to lose 15 pounds by six months post-pregnancy and regain your pre-pregnancy shape by nine months after giving birth. In addition, when you follow the 10-minute prescribed workouts in my program, you will gain back the muscle tone in your tummy area as you gradually *lose that baby fat!* (Instead of being squishy and saggy.)

" I've always had a high metabolism and I can eat whatever I want. "

"I was the one in high school everyone called the string bean. I've always been able to eat anything I want, and I never gain weight. I'm sure it will be the same after having my baby, and the weight will come off without exercise, right?"

The answer to your question is not whether the weight will come off without exercising (which is very unlikely due to the stretching and expanding of the hips during pregnancy) but the simple fact that you will need to tone and tighten the areas that were stretched out while carrying your baby for nine months. Studies show that the efforts women make during pregnancy to eat right and take care of themselves usually are not continued after the birth. In fact, a woman's weight may actually get worse compared with her pre-pregnancy weight if she doesn't take care of herself during the initial post-pregnancy period. I could sit here all day and quote statistics about why you should exercise to regain your shape after having a baby, but the real problem here is that you are setting yourself up for an unhealthy lifestyle by not exercising and you are putting yourself at risk of developing high blood pressure and other illnesses like Type II diabetes later on in life. Increasing your circulation and energy level are just a few of the benefits that you will notice immediately when you get started on my program. In addition, taking good care of yourself now as a preventative measure for the many, many years to come will not only help you feel good about yourself today, but will also help you stay in shape in case the day arrives when you decide to have another baby.

" I can't afford to join a gym. "

> "Money is really tight because I didn't go back to work after having my baby. I know my husband wants me to join a gym but we just can't afford it."

I have the answer for you: in-home workouts! Without leaving your house and without the hassle of packing everything up and putting it in your car to get to the gym (baby included), you can get all the exercise you need when you follow my *Lose That Baby Fat!* program. Gyms are great for chatting with other moms but you can do that by joining a walking group in your neighborhood or starting one yourself and incorporating the walking program I offer in this book. *You* can actually be the one to motivate others within your group of friends with my simple and easy-to-follow walking plan that begins as soon as the doctor gives you the go-ahead to begin exercising and continues for the first twelve weeks post-pregnancy. After that, you'll begin to follow the 10-minute workouts while the baby's asleep or in a bouncy seat (I found it so handy!). And as your baby gets bigger and falls into a regular napping schedule (i.e., dozes off in the car) you can increase the intensity of each 10-minute workout simply by increasing the resistance. It doesn't take a monthly fee to do all that at home and you'll start seeing improvements within a few short weeks.

" I have to go back to work. "

"I only have six weeks of maternity leave before I have to go back to work. I am thankful for the time I have now to spend with my newborn. But once I go back to the office, I don't know how I'll have time to exercise."

When it comes to exercise, many of us make the mistake of thinking, "If I can't exercise for a full hour every day, why bother at all?" This all-or-nothing approach is a sure way *not* to reach your goals. You need to learn how to get the most out of your time to lose weight and get fit, which is exactly what my program offers. The trick is to use whatever little time you do have to your best advantage. And since you are a working mom, you truly know the meaning of "multi-tasking." This means doing the things you already know how to do: walking more often, taking the stairs, standing up every now and then to move around, replacing your office chair with an exercise ball and so on. However, you still need more than that. One way to get your workout time in is to break up workouts into short segments throughout the day: 5 minutes here, 10 minutes there . . . it all adds up and that is why I devised a program that allows you to accomplish a lot in a little amount of time. In this case, the old saying really does apply: a little effort goes a long way!

" I had my baby in the winter. It's too cold outside to exercise! "

"My son was born when it was cold and snowy outside, so I'm really enjoying layering the clothes on and bundling up. I can just wait until the weather gets better before I start exercising."

It can be tough to get started when it's cold outside (although I'm sure you've been told how good fresh air is for newborns). However, I offer an easy-to-follow program that you can do *in your home*, which will not only solve your dilemma but get you back on track to feeling good in no time. Although my program begins with walking to rev up the circulation and get your heart pumping, I also offer a stretching program in Chapter 2 that can be done as soon as you feel ready (six weeks post-pregnancy) to help kick in that old metabolism and burn calories. So the good news is whether it's snowing, raining, or hailing outside, you can do my 10-minute prescribed workouts and gradually beat those winter blues until those sunny days reappear!

As you can see by the excuses offered by our reader moms, many women think getting back in shape after having a baby has to be both painstaking and time-consuming. But as you read the responses, you can see for yourself the program I offer is both easy and time-saving, which makes it accessible for everyone, no matter what her excuse may be! In addition, statistics show that the majority of woman who don't begin exercising as soon as they feel up to it after birth will be 10 pounds overweight by the end of the first year post-pregnancy. Add this to the notion of going into a second or third pregnancy and a slowing metabolism due to the aging process and as you can see, you're setting yourself up for failure by not starting early.

START EARLY AND SET REALISTIC GOALS

It's quite simple, really—the best time to shed post-pregnancy pounds is within the first six months after having a baby. It may be accomplished if you wait longer, but it will be more difficult as time goes on to lose that baby fat!

Unfortunately, most women I know think they can lose a lot of weight quickly but this just isn't true. You've probably heard the saying, "nine months up, nine months down," and there is a lot of truth to that. Your body put weight on slowly over a nine-month period to provide for your growing baby, so it isn't realistic to expect to lose those extra pounds over a shorter period of time. The average woman does not drop her baby weight overnight. Yes, the first 12 to 15 and sometimes even 20 pounds can drop off within the first three weeks after giving birth, from the weight of the placenta, the weight of the baby and the extra fluids your body was storing. However, as your body begins to adjust to all the hormonal changes that take place post-pregnancy, the remaining additional pounds tend to stick around.

So what is realistic at this stage in the game? I have found that losing 2 pounds a week is realistic and safe (if you're breast-feeding, it's 2 ½ pounds a month). Two pounds a week ensures that the skin retracts or tightens and doesn't sag. And if you gained more than 35 pounds while you were pregnant, you will need to allow an extra month of exercising and eating less or portion control for each additional 5 pounds of weight that you gained. So if you gained 45 pounds, you should achieve your goal and regain your pre-pregnancy weight around Month 10 of this program. It sounds a bit scientific but you really can chart your progress and see a difference when you break down your fitness goals in the simple month-by-month format that I offer in this book.

Most important of all, keep in mind that the ultimate goal of the *Lose That Baby Fat!* program is not only to lose the baby weight but also to tone and tighten the areas that were stretched out during pregnancy and delivery—to lose that kangaroo pouch around the middle or jiggly area that just seems weird and somehow out of place!

DON'T PUT YOUR WEIGHT LOSS GOALS LAST

Once you have a baby, your life will change forever, that's for sure. And it will be difficult to fit it all in: doing laundry, making meals, providing care for your other children (husband, ha!), going back to work, and—let's not forget—working out and eating right! Whew! However, a new mommy can't put her own needs last because she will be the one who has to have the stamina and energy to care for her new baby. So what are you waiting for? After you have your doctor's okay, get ready to go! But first, check the list below to see if you measure up before getting started.

The Rules: Fitness Guidelines

Here's what you've been waiting for—the rules or my top ten list. Follow these to a T and you'll be ready to get started in no time!

1. GIVE YOURSELF FOUR TO SIX WEEKS: In general, most moms should give themselves up to four to six weeks following delivery to recover. The American College of Obstetricians and Gynecologists reminds new moms that many of the changes that took place during pregnancy will persist for four to six weeks following birth, so you should resume exercise gradually. Those who have had a Cesarean section or medical complications may need additional time to heal.

2. HAVE A SNACK: It's always a good idea to have a high protein and carbohydrate snack an hour or so before exercise. To keep up your energy and your blood sugar steady, have a snack every two to three hours. Your snack should include calcium rich products like yogurt and cheese to replace your energy after the birth and help with osteoporosis. Of course, you don't want to eat a three-course meal before exercising, but choosing something light and healthy will help you get through your workout a lot easier.

3. DRINK WATER, WATER, WATER: Keep a water bottle handy and drink frequently. You need additional fluids when breast-feeding and when exercising. Dehydration can also make you feel drained and tired, so drink at least eight to twelve glasses of water a day.

4. STAY CENTERED: Listen to your body and slow down or rest when you feel out of breath or uncomfortable. Increasing your exercise time and intensity too quickly sets you up for injury.

5. TAKE A SHORT NAP: A 15-minute power nap will help to restore your energy level and restore your brainpower. Even if you don't fall asleep, just resting your mind and body will help you make it through the day a little bit easier.

6. TRY BREAST-FEEDING: Breast-feeding affects your metabolism in many different ways. Yes, breast-feeding does burn 500 extra calories a day as I mentioned

earlier, but it also keeps the "mama fat" hanging on for some of us. You need to take this into consideration and be realistic about how and when the weight will actually come off when breast-feeding. Every woman's body is different and therefore will respond in a different way. I found that I could not take off that last 5 pounds until I stopped breast-feeding, whereas my best friend gained 15 pounds when she stopped. It always helps to be prepared in advance for weight changes and hormone fluctuations so you can adjust your workout accordingly.

7. USE A HEART RATE MONITOR: Using a heart rate monitor (see Appendix for product information) makes a lot of sense for new moms because first of all, you don't have a lot of free time, and you really need to

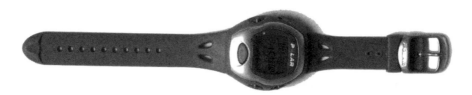

maximize the time you do have for working out. For example, a brisk-paced walk of 30 minutes using your target heart rate as a gauge for losing weight is better than a full-out run.

However, according to the U.S. Department of Health and Human Services, less than 10 percent of the population exercises three or more times a week at a level vigorous enough to improve cardiovascular fitness. Six-time Iron Man champion Dave Scott said of heart rate monitors, "Every question I ever had about exercise or training was answered when I bought, and began using, a heart rate monitor." Your heart is the most accurate measure of how hard you are working while exercising and at rest. Look at it as a personal coach of sorts that "monitors" you during your workouts. Most monitors have high and low signals or alarms that will sound if you are exercising too hard or not hard enough. They are as easy to read as a wristwatch, and usually come with a chart showing how to find the perfect training range for you.

8. KEEP TAKING PRENATAL VITAMINS: Taking prenatal vitamins is a great way to help keep up your stamina and give you the encrgy and essential vitamins and minerals you will need after having a baby. A lot of women make the mistake of thinking that after giving birth their body chemistry will go right back to where it was before the baby, which isn't true—it takes time! A woman's hair tends to fall out and become thinner the first six months after birth. Taking prenatal vitamins will prevent it from falling out at such a fast rate. Also, if you are breast-feeding, prenatal vitamins will help to supply the additional nutrients your body needs.

9. ENLIST THE HELP OF OTHERS: Whether it's a friend, relative or another mom you met in a Mommy and Me group, getting someone to watch your baby for a few hours a

week can give you that much-needed break so you can recharge your body and mind. Just don't feel you have to plan something extra special on that day off or go overboard and try to do too much—keeping it simple by seeing a movie, getting a much-needed manicure and pedicure, or simply grabbing a bite while you catch up on the latest happenings in the news, will leave you feeling refreshed and ready to face yet another day of baby challenges.

10. GIVE IN ONCE IN A WHILE: As with any new workout program, at some point along the way you're bound to take one step forward, two steps back. Or is it two steps forward, one step back? Whatever the case may be, it's important to allow yourself to take a few days off to give your body a rest. Resting in between workouts for forty-eight hours is just as important as boosting your energy level by working up a good sweat. Pushing yourself to the limit every time will just leave you tired and depleted so be good to yourself and listen to your body.

A WORD ABOUT YOUR CLOTHING!

Here's another shorter list of how and why dressing the part can be just as important as getting started in the first place.

1. GET NEW SHOES: Your feet may have increased up to a full size following pregnancy! So make sure your exercise shoes fit properly. Don't squeeze your feet into too-

small shoes—it can cause chronic foot problems. Plus, nothing seems to get us ladies more excited than slipping into something new. Shoes are a great motivator and investment when it comes to working out.

2. GET A SUPPORT BRA OR TWO: Find a bra that provides support without chafing or discomfort. Some nursing moms find that wearing two exercise bras provides comfortable support.

3. WEAR A GIRDLE: Oh, yeah . . . a tummy trimmer, girdle, or shaper—whatever you want to call it—can be very effective in keeping it all together and can help squeeze out some of the extra water weight that the body has retained (see Appendix for product information). It

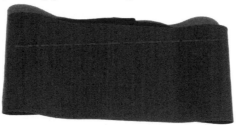

definitely helps reshape the hips and tummy area, and brings awareness to the abdominal area that hasn't been in use for nine months. When women get liposuction, they have to wear a trimmer or girdle for the first four to six weeks to help the new area that has been reshaped actually hold its new shape. The same goes for the post-pregnancy tummy that needs all the help it can get to reduce the jiggly appearance.

4. DON'T CHANGE YOUR WARDROBE: The worst advice I received after having my baby was to throw away my old jeans because they'd never fit again. I'm so glad I didn't because it felt great when I was able to fit back into them. Do not go out and buy all new clothes right after having a baby. With the exception of a few new tops or a pair of slacks, it is imperative that you don't buy any new "bigger sized" clothes. I know all of us have had that wonderful feeling of being able to fit into an old pair of jeans. That feeling can be a great motivator when you're trying to lose weight. I am a big believer in throwing away the scale and using clothes and sizes to determine where your weight really is. When the body gains muscle through effectively working out, the muscle weighs more than fat, so it does cause temporary weight gain on the scale. However, since bigger muscles burn more fat, you will start to see results right away in inches rather than on the scale. In fact, holding on to your old jeans and trying them on along the way can prove to be very inspiring when you finally do fit into those skinny jeans . . . and you will!

GATHERING YOUR GEAR

Now that you know where you stand in terms of being physically ready to begin working out, check the list below to see what equipment you'll need as you start moving through the following chapters in this book and getting in the best shape of your life! (Please note that all of the equipment listed below is inexpensive, easy to use, and can be found in the Appendix under product information).

EXERCISE BALL: Look for anti-burst or burst resistant and latex-free in the following sizes:

HEIGHT	BALL SIZE
48" to 5'3"	55cm ball
5'4" to 6'	65cm ball
6'0 and up	75cm ball

The best way to tell whether or not your new ball is the correct height is to sit on it. The recommended height allows you to bend your knees at a 90-degree angle when you're sitting on the ball and your feet are flat on the floor. This angle allows your hips to be level or slightly higher than your knees.

Check the instructions for inflating your ball when you purchase it. Make sure to always keep it filled to the proper level with air to ensure you are getting the best workout possible.

RESISTANCE BANDS:

Resistance bands are great because they're very inexpensive and easier to use than weights. The main thing to look for when

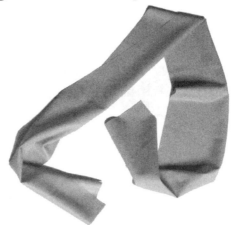

purchasing resistance bands are the varying levels of resistance (light, medium, and heavy) and the correct length. A band that is 5- or 5 ½-feet-long is the easiest to use and can move in all directions around your ball so you'll have the resistance you need wherever you move.

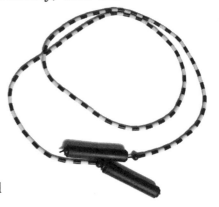

JUMP ROPE: Jumping rope (as you will soon find out) is a quick and easy way to reduce cellulite and burn a lot of calories by boosting your metabolism and revving up your circulation. Jumping rope also tones muscles throughout your entire body, upper and lower, and increases your endurance, which is essential for new moms. Plus you only need a small area (around 3 feet by 4 feet) so you can do it anywhere or anytime.

PEDOMETER: Pedometers are coming back in a big way and for a very good reason—they work! A pedometer counts the steps you take and has other uses like counting calories and measuring distance. All you have to do is attach one to your waist and aim

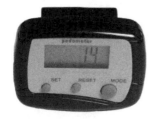

for the recommended 6,000 to 10,000 steps a day. (See Chapter 2 to learn how the *Lose That Baby Fat!* walking and stretching exercises meets that goal.)

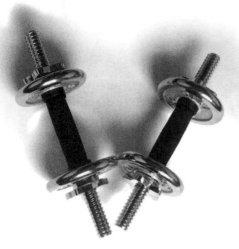

HAND WEIGHTS: When choosing your hand weights or dumbbells, pick only the amount of weight that will allow you to do ten to twelve repetitions resulting in your muscles feeling fatigued. Building lean muscle mass during your 10-minute workouts is the key to toning up and losing weight fast. For most women, ten to fifteen pounds is a good amount of weight to use.

EASING INTO EXERCISE

Equipment Needed: Just you.

Yay! You made it through delivery and now are ready to begin your very first exercise that will help strengthen and tone the pelvic floor otherwise known as the Kegel muscles. Kegel muscles are the muscles that line the inner walls of the vagina and pelvis and are responsible for controlling the flow of urine, resulting in bladder control. Because you will still look six months pregnant right after having a baby, working your Kegel muscles will help tremendously after giving birth to not only regain bladder control (which you'll soon find out is no easy feat when you sneeze!) but also help return your uterus to its pre-pregnancy size.

Kegel exercises are easy and safe to do soon after delivery and can be done while you're taking a warm bath, sitting in a chair or lying in bed. To strengthen the kegel muscles, follow these simple and easy steps:

1. Lie on the floor or sit comfortably in a chair with your knees together.

   To help you feel the muscles you are working, make sure your feet are flat on the floor.

2. Tense the same muscles in the vagina that you would use to keep from urinating (Kegel muscles).

   Make sure the rest of your body stays relaxed as you tense **only** your Kegel muscles.

3. Hold for five seconds or longer before releasing your Kegel muscles and resting.

   For best results, perform kegel exercises twice a day for 3 to 5 minutes each time or 20 to 30 repetitions.

AND FINALLY

Although your body may seem like a bit of a stranger to you, there are so many other important things to focus on right now. Of course, the most important one would be your baby.

And don't forget to pat yourself on the back just for wanting to get up and go outside. It's always inspiring to me when I see a new mom walking her newborn in a stroller or a carrier. I think about how time-consuming it can be just to get out of the house in the first place, and about all the things you need to tote along with you. The little strides you make throughout the day now will turn into big strides as you look back. And as everybody told me time after time (which I did find annoying), it goes by so fast. So enjoy your time in the "baby cave" as many new moms call it, because before you know it, you'll be chasing your toddler around the house and you'll really need those running shoes!

2

The First 6 to 8 Weeks After Birth: Walking and Stretching

How Your Body May Look:
Still fitting into your maternity clothes

How You May Be Feeling:
Tired and a bit "foggy" from sleep deprivation

How Much Weight You Will Have Lost:
Approximately 12 to 15 pounds from delivery

Equipment Needed:
A stroller or Baby Bjorn–type carrier
and an exercise ball for stretching

"

After I had my son Joey, the hardest part about getting back into shape was getting started. It was overwhelming enough just taking my newborn out of the house on a simple errand, let alone finding a way to go work out! Before I became pregnant, I was very active and kept myself in good shape. I gained about 35 pounds during my pregnancy, which I realize isn't all that much but it was still scary to see the scale climb. After Joey was born, the first 13 pounds came off in a blink. The next 7 pounds came off with very little effort so I was extremely happy. I was breast-feeding, which may have helped because nursing apparently burns a lot of calories. The last 10 pounds were a different story! I had to buckle down, get back to a regular workout routine and eat less. It was difficult to figure out a way to work out with my baby. I couldn't just run off to a yoga class or jump on the treadmill whenever I pleased. The best solution I found was walking. Not a leisurely stroll but a well-paced power walk for at least twenty minutes. The great thing about walking is you just put your baby in the stroller and go! A helpful tool is a heart rate monitor. Walking for health is important but I wanted to burn calories! The monitor allows you to make sure you are in your target heart range, which is the fat burning zone. Finding other moms to walk with helps, too. Chatting and socializing with a friend makes it more fun! **"**

—Kelly Bonanno, mother of two-year-old Joey and expecting number two

● ● ○ ○ ○ ○

○ ○ ○ ○ ○ ○

YES, I REMEMBER IT WELL MYSELF. Six weeks after giving birth to my daughter Bella, I was feeling pretty good about myself and ready to venture out in my little black dress. Black always works well on anybody in any situation, right? Or so I thought until I saw my five-year-old niece and she told me that I "looked like I still had a baby in my tummy." Well, I did look like a stranger when I caught my reflection in the mirror, but I didn't think it was *that* obvious.

Enter walking. Walking is my recommended primary exercise during the first six to twelve weeks after delivery because walking is the best way to decrease fatigue from not sleeping and to increase your energy level. Walking also helps to stretch out the hip muscles while improving muscle tone in the pelvic floor and increasing circulation. Typically, new moms are given the green light to begin exercising by their doctor after their six-week checkup. Moms who have had a Cesarean section usually need to wait a bit longer. After the doctor gives you the okay to begin exercising, walking will be the most beneficial to your body, as you'll need to avoid heavy lifting and climbing stairs for the first twelve weeks.

BREAK UP YOUR WALKING ROUTINE

The most common complaint I hear from women is that they "don't have enough time to work out," meaning they don't have a full hour. Well, this may come as a surprise to you *but* you don't need an entire hour to get your daily exercise and burn calories because it's the accumulation of what you're doing throughout the entire day that really matters. Plus breaking up your workouts into shorter segments makes them more convenient and boosts your metabolism by getting your heart rate up *twice* in one day. So by doing two shorter walks rather than trying to fit it all into one long walk, you are providing yourself with a workable routine that can easily be fit into your busy schedule. Of course, if you find yourself walking longer than ten minutes at a time, that's great! But remember to keep it simple and not overdo it so you can stick to the twice-daily program in this chapter. Before you get started, take the time to read the following tips to make your walks go a little smoother.

PICK A ROUTE YOU CAN FOLLOW EVERY DAY: Starting right outside your front door is easier than packing everything up and lugging it in and out of the car repeatedly (and when you're aiming for ten minutes of walking, it makes a lot more sense). Choosing a neighborhood coffee shop, park, school, or any other destination within walking distance will help. And if you're returning to work, you're actually at an advantage because you won't have your baby to schedule things around so you can use your lunch hour to quickly change into your walking shoes and walk to lunch. After twelve weeks post-pregnancy, you'll be able to add stairs, which you'll find at the park or at the office (hopefully you're on the fifth floor and not the tenth) that will help strengthen your abdominals and get your heart pumping even more.

TIME YOUR WALKS: Before you leave the house you'll want to be sure and throw on the kitchen timer, check the clock, or wear a sports watch because you need to know exactly how long your walks are from beginning to end. Timing your daily walks in this manner will help you keep track of your progress as you gain stamina and endurance along the way.

TRY A PEDOMETER: As I mentioned in Chapter 1, a pedo-meter measures each step you take and is a great way to tell how far you've walked. For the walking program prescribed in this chapter, you will be walking a total of two miles a day. Because each mile is equal to 2,000 steps, you will be taking a total of 4,000 steps during your twice-daily 10-minute walks. And because the average adult takes 6,000 steps throughout the day during regular activity, you've just met the goal of the recommended 10,000 steps a day for fitness.

USE THE RIGHT EQUIPMENT: You'll want to use a light-weight but sturdy stroller for your walking program just in case you hit any bumps or cracks (I cover baby joggers later in this book because they are usually reserved for babies that are closer to twelve months old and up to 50 pounds). If you are going to use a front-style carrier for your baby such as a Baby Bjorn, which will allow you to swing your arms a bit, the weight requirements are 8 to 25 pounds. However, most people stop using them when the baby reaches around 20 pounds because the heavier weight causes pulling in the shoulders and strain in the upper back.

GO FOR A HEART RATE MONITOR: Using a heart rate monitor is a great way to quickly identify your fat burning zone (between 60 and 80 percent of your maximum heart rate) and get the exact number of calories you're burning during your workout. If you want to figure out your target heart rate, you subtract your age from 220 then multiply anywhere between .6 (60 percent) and .8 (80 percent) to find out when you are in your fat burning zone. Working above your 80-percent target heart rate would put you in the cardiovascular training range, which is not what we're trying to achieve for this walking program.

WALKING PROGRAM

The following walking program breaks the first six to eight weeks after birth into three different intervals so you can gradually increase the intensity of your walks as you gain strength and stamina. Each interval burns approximately

75 calories in 10 minutes so you will be burning a total of 150 calories by doing the twice-daily walks (which equals 20 minutes on the elliptical trainer at the gym) I prescribe in this chapter. In addition, if you add the stretches at the end of this chapter right after your walks, you will be burning an additional 150 calories, which gives you a total of 300 calories burned in one day—a great goal for where you are right now post-pregnancy!

If you're using a baby stroller for walking, you'll want to tuck your butt under and tighten your tummy as you stride along. You'll also want to keep your elbows in and bent to keep the stroller from getting too far out in front of your body. As the old saying goes, "Make sure you're walking the dog and the dog's not walking you!" If you're using a front-style carrier to hold the baby for your walks, remember to pump your arms as you keep your elbows in and close to your body. This will allow you to maintain a strong and steady pace without losing your form.

> SIX WEEKS AFTER BIRTH: Start out walking in the morning using a slow pace and gradually work up to a steady brisk pace for 10 minutes. As you finish your walk, return to the slower pace you started out with to cool your body down properly. Repeat this 10-minute walking exercise later on in the day, possibly after dinner for the best results.

> SEVEN WEEKS AFTER BIRTH: The following walking intervals work best when you're able to time them with a sports watch (although you can approximate

the times if you need to). Start out by walking one minute fast, then proceed to three minutes slow, one minute fast, three minutes slow, one minute fast, and end with one minute slow. The constant change in pace this walking exercise provides will increase and decrease your heart rate so you'll be able to get a better fat burning workout in a shorter period of time. Repeat the 1/3,1/3,1/1 intervals later in the day.

EIGHT WEEKS AFTER BIRTH: You are now ready to increase the duration of your walks to one long walk consisting of 20 minutes. For this walking exercise, it's best to start out with an accelerated pace and end with a slower pace to allow your body to cool down properly. Allow enough time at the end of your walk when your muscles are warm and ready to go for the stretching routine prescribed in this chapter.

STRETCHING ROUTINE ON THE BALL

Adding a few stretches right after walking will not only in-crease your flexibility but will also burn additional calories. I suggest trying the exercises in the following sequence because they allow you to work the body in a natural progression—from top to bottom. You will need an exercise ball to do the following stretches.

The Upper Body Stretch

The upper body stretch will loosen the muscles in your upper back as you let your upper body and arms drop toward the floor.

A. Sit on the ball with your back straight and your legs stretched out in front of you. Place your hands under your lower legs or touch your ankles, while you lean forward from your waist.

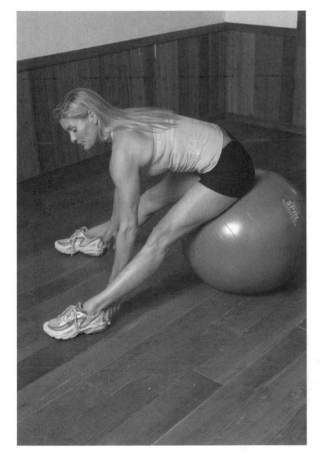

B. Place your hands on your thighs for support, then release back up to your starting position.

The Hamstring Stretch

The hamstring stretch is great to do right after your walk to stretch out the muscles in the back of your legs and increase your flexibility.

A. Sit on the ball with your weight slightly forward. Your feet will be a little wider than shoulder-width apart. Extend your right leg to one side until it's straight. With your hands on your hips, lean forward from your waist as you lower your chest down toward your right leg. Hold for a few seconds before bending your knee and rolling back up into starting position.

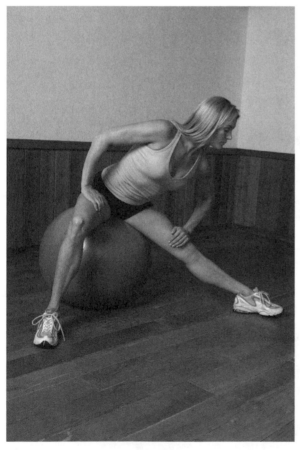

B. Repeat 3 stretches on each leg.

The Quads Stretch

The quads stretch helps stretch out the muscles in the front of your legs or thighs. Your quads or quadriceps can get pretty tight just like the hamstrings, so it's especially good to stretch these two muscle groups right after one another.

A. Lie with your tummy on the ball so it is directly under your hips. To maintain your balance place your right hand and right leg on the floor as you lift your left leg behind you. Raise your left arm up and reach behind you to grab your left ankle. Stretch the front of your leg using a gentle pulling motion. Lower your left arm and left leg to the floor before repeating on the other side.

B. Repeat 3 times on each leg.

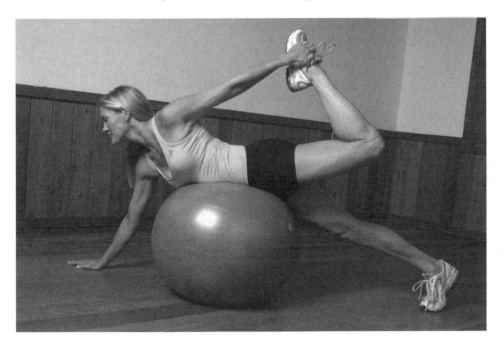

The Waist Stretch

The waist stretch lengthens out the sides of your waist by working the obliques. It helps improve your posture and gives you a longer, leaner appearance.

A. Kneel next to the ball and rest your right side or rib cage against the ball. Your right arm will be wrapped around the ball for support and your left leg will be extended out to the side. Raise your left arm over your head as you exhale, stretching the left side of your body.

B. Repeat for 5 repetitions on both sides.

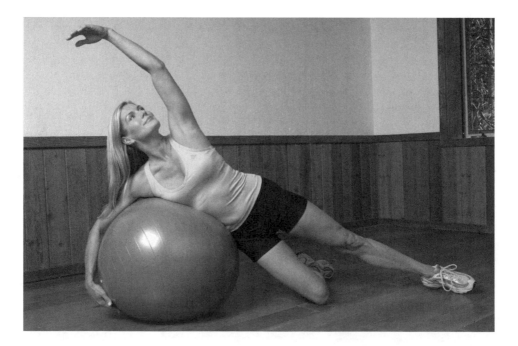

The Shoulder Stretch

This exercise is effective for stretching out the muscles in your chest and throughout the shoulders. Be sure to breathe as you place your weight on the ball to stretch out your shoulders.

A. Kneeling behind the ball, stretch both arms straight out on top of the ball. Let your eyes gaze down to the floor to keep your neck in line with your spine. Breathe and hold for a few seconds.

B. Repeat 3 times.

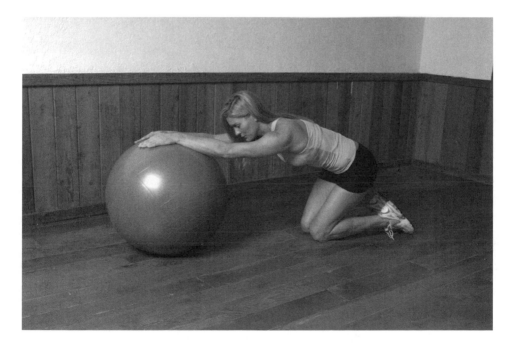

The Drape

The perfect ending to any workout is the drape exercise. And it is done exactly as it sounds—by draping your body frontward over the ball. You can rock back and forth once you get into this position to stretch out all the muscles in your back and increase your flexibility.

A. Place your tummy on the ball and drape your entire body over the ball facing down. Wrap your arms around the ball as if you were giving it a big hug as you rest your head to one side.

B. Once you feel comfortable, rest your fingertips on the floor in front of you for an extra stretch. Return to starting position and rest on your knees before repeating.

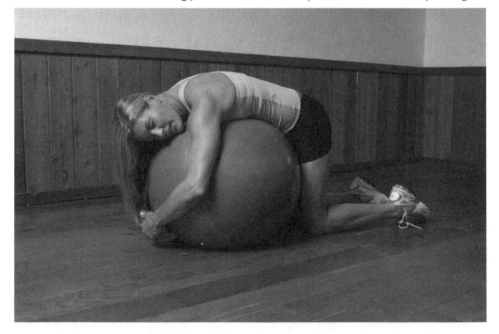

GOT REST?

By now you're starting to figure out that your baby is going to need a lot—diaper changes, constant love and attention, and sleep. But what about you? As I mentioned in Chapter 1, it's important for *you* to get rest because you are the one that will have to take care of your entire family because everybody depends on Mom, right? Ah, the pressure!

Don't worry, you'll get through the sleep deprivation—nothing lasts forever and if you sleep when the baby sleeps, you'll feel a whole lot better than trying to constantly be on the go. And don't forget your walks! They will help you feel refreshed and revitalized plus—isn't it great how they get your baby to sleep?

3

Three Months After Birth: Phenomenal Abdominals

How Your Body May Look:
Poochy around the middle

How You May Be Feeling:
Thinking twice about continuing with breast-feeding. Experiencing a returning period if you never breast-fed.

How Much Weight You May Have Lost:
Another 7 to 10 pounds from uterine involution

Equipment Needed:
Exercise ball

"

Having my first two girls so close together really took its toll on my body. It wasn't so much the weight because I knew I would probably lose that just like I did with my first—but it was the EXTRA FOLDS of skin around my stomach that really scared me! I guess it only makes sense that after giving birth you're going to look different, but I really have to work hard now to keep my stomach pulled in. I think it really helps to know this before you have a baby so you can be prepared for what your stomach is going to look like afterwards—an empty kangaroo pouch! **"**

—Laura Stanley, mother of nine-year-old Dara, six-year-old Danielle, and four-year-old Dayna Rey

● ● ● ○ ○ ○

○ ○ ○ ○ ○ ○

"A BABY SHOULD CHANGE YOUR LIFE, NOT YOUR BODY." What idiot said that? I doubt they ever had a baby . . . or two or three! At three months after giving birth, you might notice that your tummy looks like a deflated balloon. And, as you've probably heard the saying: "nine months up, nine months down," you now know that it's true! Slowly but surely you *will* see the tone return to your abdominal area, but it will take work. All new moms can benefit from exercises that strengthen their pelvic floor and abdominal muscles. These muscles, which were weakened during pregnancy, need specific work to increase tone and to prevent the development of incontinence and back problems.

This chapter contains some of the best exercises you can do to help get back in touch with your abdominal muscles and help safely target and strengthen the muscles in the pelvic floor. After doing a warm-up consisting of walking or calisthenics to help get your blood flowing and your heart pumping, I suggest picking four of the following exercises that can be done safely and easily three to four times a week to start. As you begin to build a stronger core and improve your abdominal strength, try adding a few more of the exercises in this chapter to provide you with a more challenging workout.

The Ball Pulldown

This beginner exercise allows you to gently work the abdominal muscles by bringing the ball in to meet your knees.

A. Lie on your back with your knees bent and your feet flat on the floor. Raise the ball above your head.

B. Exhale as you bring the ball to meet your knees. Your upper body and lower back must remain on the floor at all times.

C. Repeat 10 to 12 repetitions.

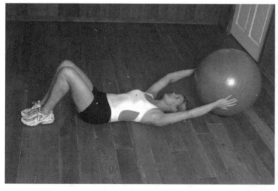

A.

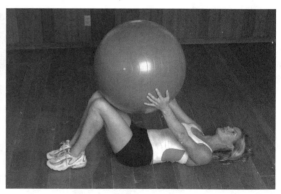

B.

The Bicycle with the Ball

This conventional bicycle exercise becomes even more effective when you use the ball because it targets the lower abdominal muscles each time you lengthen out your legs.

A. Lie flat on your back with your knees bent and your feet flat on the floor. Raise the ball above your head. Bring one knee in at a time to meet the ball as you extend the opposite leg out straight and off the floor.

B. Exhale as you straighten each leg out and inhale as you bring each knee in toward your chest.

C. Repeat 10 to 12 repetitions.

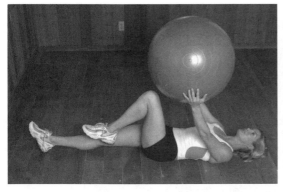

A.

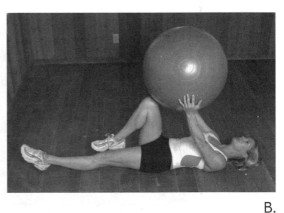

B.

The Abdominal Crunch

You've probably done a lot of sit-ups in your lifetime and that is exactly what the abdominal crunch is—only it's done on the ball. For this exercise, you want to make sure you are halfway between a sitting and lying position with your lower back supported by the ball.

A. Sit on the ball with your feet shoulder-width apart and your knees at a 90-degree angle. Slowly walk your feet out in front of you until your lower back is on the ball.

B. With your hands behind your head and your elbows bent out to the sides, curl your body up into a sitting position. Slowly roll back down onto the ball, one vertebrae at a time.

C. Repeat for 10 to 12 repetitions.

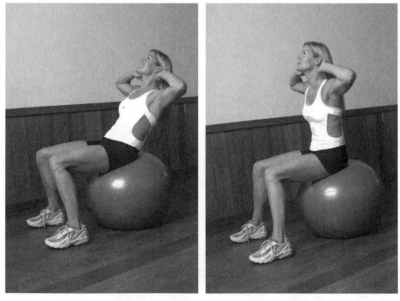

A.   B.

The Reverse Curl

When you bring your upper body to meet your lower body, otherwise known as a reverse curl, you are really working your tummy area. This is a very effective exercise for targeting the abs!

A. Lie with your back flat on the floor and place your legs on the ball.

B. As you tighten your tummy, grasp the ball between your lower legs or calves and pull it toward you, lifting the ball from the floor. Slowly lift your shoulders from the floor bringing your shoulders toward your knees. Hold for a few seconds, and then slowly roll your shoulders back to the floor and release the ball.

C. Repeat for 10 repetitions.

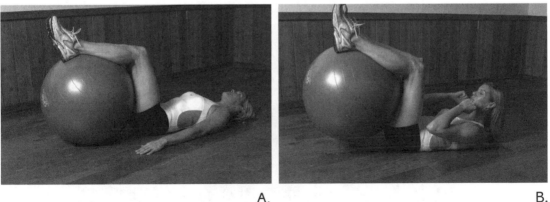

A.   B.

The Waist Trimmer

I really see a difference in my waist when I do this exercise! The waist trimmer also works the shoulders when you move them side-to-side across your body. And everyone knows that broader shoulders make the waist appear smaller, right?

A. Lie with your back on the ball and your knees bent at a 90-degree angle. Your shoulders will not touch the ball, so they're free to move from side to side.

B. Bring your arms to your chest and rest your chin on your hands. Starting with your right shoulder, contract your abdominal muscles as you slowly lift and turn your body toward your left hip. Hold for a few seconds, and then slowly lower your body to the starting position. Slowly lift your left shoulder as you contract your abdominal muscles and turn your body toward your right hip.

C. Alternate right and left side lifts for 10 to 12 repetitions.

A.

B.

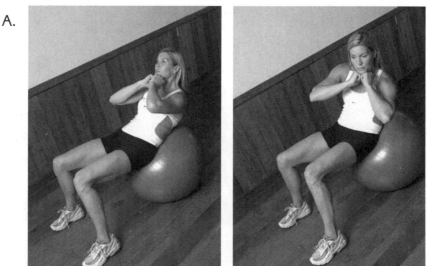

The Roll Away

The roll away strengthens the entire core of your body and tightens the deep abdominal muscles that are harder to target. It may take a few tries to get this one right!

A. Kneeling in front of the ball, place the palms of your hands on the ball at arm's length.

B. Contract your abdominal muscles and tuck in your butt, while rolling the ball away from you slightly so that your forearms rest on the ball. Hold for a few seconds before returning to starting position.

C. Repeat 10 repetitions.

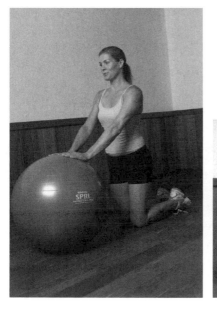

A.

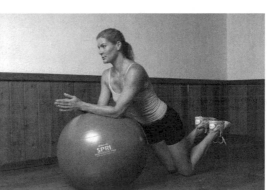

B.

The Abdominal Tuck

The abdominal tuck is great for strengthening your tummy and your upper body because you perform it in the push-up position. This exercise is good for toning the entire body.

A. Lie with the ball under your stomach and roll forward until the ball rests under your shins.

B. Pull the ball in using your hips, and slowly tuck your knees into your chest. Hold for a few seconds, then slowly extend your legs back out into the starting position.

C. Repeat 10 repetitions.

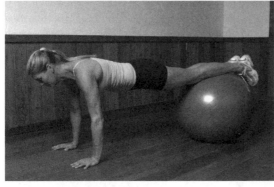
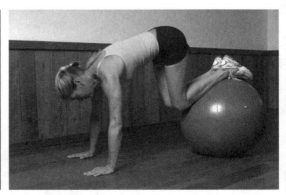

A.   B.

The Ball Exchange

This is my absolute favorite exercise for training your core. It's also good for teaching hand-and-eye coordination, as you'll see when you start passing the ball back and forth between your arms and legs.

A. Lie on your back making sure your lower back is pressed down. Holding the ball, extend your arms and the ball directly above your head on the floor.

A.

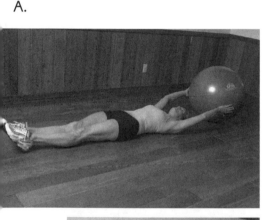

B. Raise your arms and legs up to meet at a 90-degree angle above your torso.

C. Exchange the ball by grasping it between your legs then bring the ball back down to the floor.

D. Continue exchanging the ball 10 to 12 times.

B.

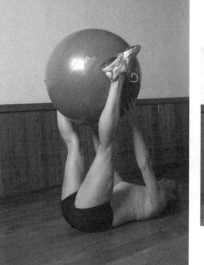

C.

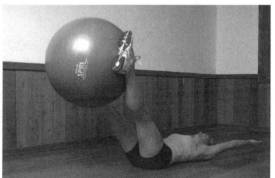

ROME WASN'T BUILT IN A DAY AND NEITHER WERE YOU!

By now you're probably figuring out that it's going to take some time to get your body back. After all, it did take you nine months to lose it, right? And as I mentioned in Chapter 1, even if you are one of the lucky few whose weight drops right off, your tummy may look like a deflated balloon, a wrinkly wallet, an accordion, or some other musical instrument . . . you get the point.

It's not really about the weight, is it? And it's not all about having a flat tummy. It's about feeling good about yourself and having the energy to do it all—feedings, diaper changes, laundry, making dinner, etc. So keep in mind, you will bounce back . . . it just takes time! And be patient—as I mentioned before, *Rome wasn't built in a day.*

4

Four Months After Birth: Shapely Arms and Chest

How Your Body May Be Looking:
Flabby arms or loss of muscle tone throughout your chest and upper body

What You May Be Experiencing:
Hair loss

How You May Be Feeling:
Hormonally challenged

Equipment Needed:
Resistance band and an exercise ball

"

Boy, did I have the most beautiful hair when I was pregnant! For the first time in my life, everybody commented on how long and shiny my hair was and I even liked it myself. Then I had my first baby and right around the third month or so, my hair started falling out! At first I thought something was wrong with my thyroid because that's what my family said it might be, but then I soon found out from my doctor that it's quite common to lose your hair from all the hormones settling down after childbirth and returning to normal. It did grow back and that made me happy until I had my second baby, and had to go through it all over again. I guess motherhood really is about experiencing it all—the good and the bad. But I wouldn't trade it for the world; it's the best! **"**

—Adele Clarkson, mother of two-year-old David, and four-year-old Trina

● ● ● ● ○ ○

○ ○ ○ ○ ○ ○

IS YOUR HAIR FALLING OUT? If you answered "yes," don't worry; you're right on schedule, because this is around the time your hormones start to settle back in and your hair starts falling out! Yes, it happens to everyone who has a baby and yes, it's just part of the overall process. The good news is, your hair will grow back. The bad news is, it's annoying and probably all over your bathroom. Mine clogged up the shower so the plumber had to come out and actually asked me, "Are you losing your hair?" It was embarrassing, but I lived through it and so will you!

As far as your body goes, that baby sure is getting heavy, isn't it? And you're going to need strong arms to lift not only the baby, but also the baby carrier, stroller, baby bag, blankets, toys, bouncy seat, and . . . well, you get the hint. Who knew such a tiny baby would need so many things?

This chapter contains a powerful group of arm and chest exercises that you can do on the ball. You'll see faster results when you use the ball because when you sit on it, you engage your core muscles in addition to working your arms and chest. You will also need a resistance band that is long enough to move in all directions around the ball (around 5 ½ feet). Resistance bands are easier on the joints than using weights and will allow you to increase your flexibility as well as tone and tighten your arms and chest. Before you begin your workout, always start out with a short warm-up consisting of walking, biking, hiking, swimming, or calisthenics.

The Biceps Curl

This exercise strengthens and tones the muscles in your arms, making it easier for you to tote the baby around. Be sure to raise and lower your arms slowly to get the full benefit of this exercise.

A. Sit on the ball with your feet flat on the floor and your knees at a 90-degree angle. Place the band under your feet and grab the ends of the band with your hands at waist level. Your palms will be facing up toward the ceiling.

B. Slowly curl your arms and the band toward your shoulders as you keep your feet flat on the floor. Lower your arms back down to your sides in starting position. Be sure to keep your wrists straight and not bent.

C. Repeat 10 to 12 repetitions.

A.

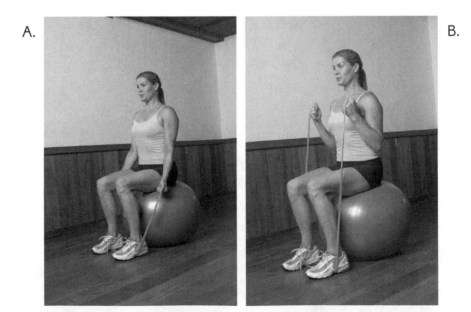

B.

The Triceps Kickback

The triceps or muscles that run along the backs of the arms can be a trouble area for most women. This exercise will help tone and tighten the triceps and work your core at the same time.

A. Sit on the ball with your knees bent at a 90-degree angle and your feet flat on the floor. Place the band under your feet and bend forward from your waist. Your hands will be at your waist with your palms facing into your body.

B. Slowly straighten your elbows and extend your arms out behind your body. Return to starting position by bending your elbows and bringing your arms back in. Make sure you maintain the slight bend in your waist.

C. Repeat 10 to 12 repetitions.

A.

B.

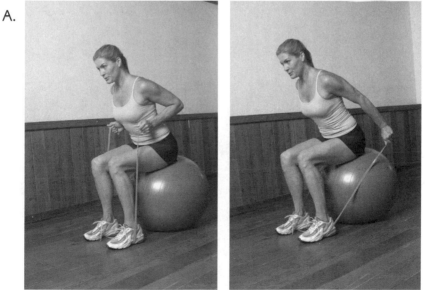

79

The Overhead Press

The overhead press works the biceps in your arms and is also great for defining and shaping the top of your shoulders.

A. Sit on the ball with your feet shoulder-width apart and place the band securely under your feet. Hold the ends of the band in your hands at shoulder level, being sure to keep your palms facing forward.

B. Straighten your arms above your head and hold for a few seconds. Slowly bring your arms back to shoulder level or starting position.

C. Repeat 10 to 12 repetitions.

A. 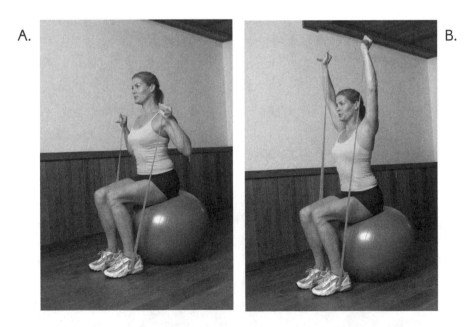 B.

The Chest Press

The chest press helps define and lift your breasts by firming up the muscles in the entire chest area.

A. Lie with your upper back and shoulders on the ball. Place the resistance band under your upper back and the ball as you hold the ends of the band in each hand. Your thighs should be parallel to the floor.

B. With your elbows bent to the sides, press your arms to the ceiling as you contract the muscles in your chest and tighten your tummy muscles. Return to starting position by relaxing your elbows back to your body and even with your shoulders.

C. Repeat 10 times.

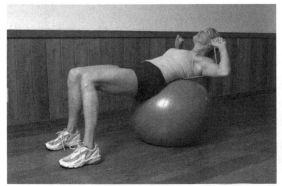

A.

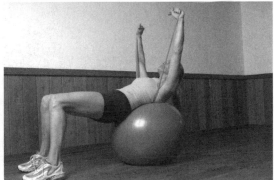

B.

The Push-Up

Nothing works and tones the chest area like a good old-fashioned push-up. And when you add the ball, you get the additional benefit of working your tummy muscles. If you have time to do only a few exercises, make sure this is one of them.

A. Lie with your belly on the ball and walk your hands forward until the ball rests under your lower legs or shins. Make sure that you keep your hands directly below your shoulders.

B. Lower your upper body toward the floor, bending the elbows out to the sides. Straighten the elbows and exhale as you press back up into starting position.

C. Repeat 10 times.

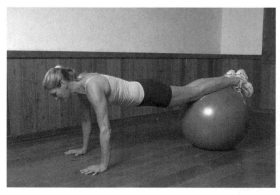

A.

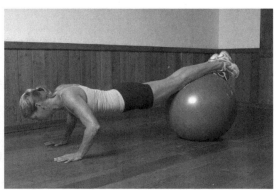

B.

VACATION TIME

Right around now, most new moms feel confident enough to take a family vacation with their newest member in tow. If you do decide to take a trip, here's a word of warning—you'll need a lot of stuff! I remember the first time I flew with my daughter and had to lug around a heavy car seat and stroller, while carrying her all at the same time. Now that takes talent! And just try taking a cruise before they're old enough to go to day camp or babysitting. That's a real treat!

Yes, it can be stressful once you discover all the supplies you'll need for yourself, your baby, your husband, and any other children in your family when you decide to take a trip. But breaking out of your routine—plus the family photos you'll get—are worth the hassle in the end. Sometimes just getting a change of scenery can do everyone in the family good, and if nothing else, you'll certainly be glad to return home once again. Just don't forget to bring along a good book for reading or exercising . . .

Five Months After Birth: Booty-Licious

How Your Body May Look:
Larger through the hips from the
stretching and expanding of pregnancy

How You May Be Feeling:
Discouraged because you don't
have your former body back yet

Equipment Needed:
Exercise ball

"

I'm a thirty-eight-year-old mom who gave birth to my second son five months ago. Luckily for me, I was blessed with the genetic ability to drop all my pregnancy weight (30 pounds) within the first month after delivery (don't hate me!); and the weight stays off as long as I breast-feed. I'm happy with my clothing size, but I definitely have a problem area: the tummy and hips! Both my boys were huge at birth (my first, Travis, was almost 12 pounds; the second, Owen, almost 11 pounds). It seems that not only have my abs given out, but also the skin on my tummy is flabby and I seem to be carrying a disproportionate amount of fat there. Plus it's so wrinkly! It looks like the stomach of a seventy-year-old! And my hips are all stretched out and that doesn't help any . . . I wonder if there's any hope for that area, or if this is a permanent change and I should just toss out all my two-piece swimsuits and my clingy T-shirts. I exercise by taking the kids out in the double jogger stroller a few times a week, but I don't have a regular routine yet. I don't have the time or the childcare available to be able to go to the gym, so I need a plan I can carry out at home, both for cardio and the tummy area. Help! **"**

—Erin Newman, mother to two-year-old Travis, and five-month-old Owen.

● ● ● ● ● ○

○ ○ ○ ○ ○ ○

HERE'S SOMETHING TO CONSIDER: It's possible to lose all your baby weight and *still* be a larger size. When things stretch out that much, they don't always go back. Your hips may never be as small as they were, and you may have extra stretched skin around your middle that no amount of dieting can possibly make go away. Don't let anyone make you feel bad about that: You've accomplished something wonderful in exchange for those small-figure "flaws"! You may not ever go back to your pre-pregnancy size, but you can tone and tighten what you've been left with. The best places to start toning are the hips and legs, since these "powerhouses" of your body are the likely location of your extra weight. This chapter contains a complete lower body workout that you can do on the ball to help tighten and tone your glutes and hips.

BOOTY BALL WORKOUT

Booty, butt, or whatever you like to call your rear view, the truth is a more pronounced *derriere* has replaced the trend of having a flat butt (*now that's good news*) and hopefully it's here to stay. The following lunges, squats, and other ball exercises will help you define your booty, giving your backside a shapelier look while simultaneously toning and tightening your hips.

87

Before you begin, you'll want to start with a warm-up to get your heart rate up slowly and increase muscle temperature. Because you are working the large muscle groups in the lower half of the body, it's important to warm them up properly by walking, biking, jogging, jumping rope (see Chapter 7), or doing calisthenics.

The Wall Lunge

This exercise combines a classic lunge position with the ball that allows you to work the muscles under your butt giving the entire area a nice lift along with some real definition.

A. With your feet hip-width, place the ball between the wall and your lower back or tailbone. Make sure you are pressing into the wall to maintain the position of the ball.

B. Step out with your right leg and lower down into a lunge position until your knee is bent at a 90-degree angle. Make sure to keep your back heel lifted on your left leg. Press yourself back up to a standing position using your butt and hamstring muscles. Repeat the movement on the other side.

C. Repeat for 10 repetitions.

A.

B.

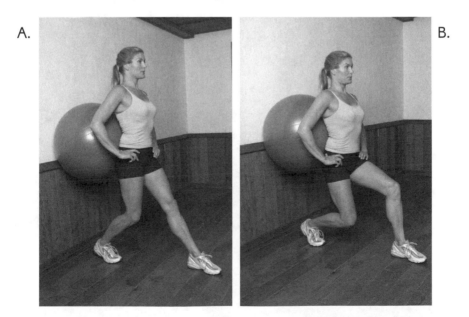

The Lunge Off the Ball

Using the ball to steady yourself as you lower down into a classic lunge position really helps strengthen your core as you work on maintaining your balance throughout this exercise.

A. With the ball to one side of your body, place your fingertips on top of the ball.

B. Step forward into a lunge position as you use the ball to maintain your balance. Hold the lunge position as you relax your body weight lower to the floor. Exhale as you straighten your leg and return to the starting position.

C. Repeat 10 times on each leg.

A. 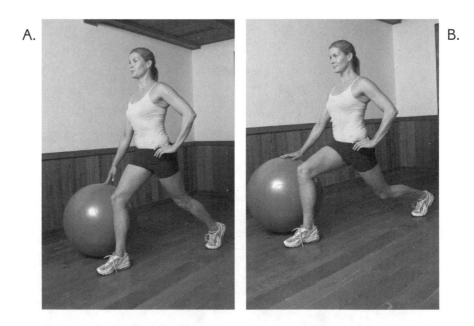 B.

The Wall Squat

You can't beat squats for working your lower body. And doing them on the ball suddenly turns a standard squatting position into a more difficult one. The wall squat is a great exercise you can do to literally work your butt off!

A. Using a wall for support, place the ball between the wall and your lower back as you walk your feet out slightly.

B. Lower down into a squatting position as if you were going to sit in a chair as you push your weight back into the ball. Make sure you press your weight into the ball for better control of the movement. Hold for a few seconds before straightening your legs.

C. Repeat for 10 to 12 repetitions.

A.

B.

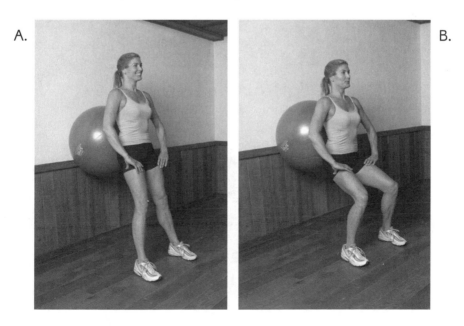

The Squat Off the Ball

This exercise combines a squat and the ball in a very simple yet effective way. By holding the ball at chest level, you are working on balance as you tighten and tone your backside.

A. Stand up tall with a straight back and bring the ball to chest level.

B. Keeping your back straight, squat down until your knees are bent at a 90-degree angle or as far as you feel comfortable. Hold for a few seconds then bring the ball down to your waist as you straighten your legs.

C. Repeat for 10 repetitions.

A. 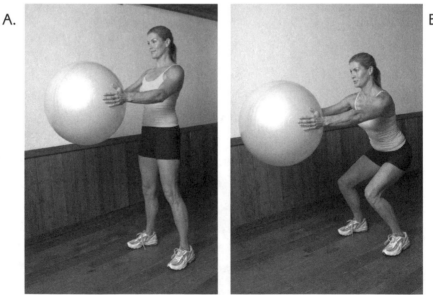 B.

The Hip Lift

This exercise uses your entire lower body to control the movement of the ball. Remember to press your body weight into the ball when you're lifting up with your hips to keep the ball steady.

A. Lie flat on the floor with your feet and ankles on top of the ball. Your arms will be alongside your body on the floor for support.

B. Pressing down into the ball with your feet to maintain your balance, exhale as you raise your hips and pelvis toward the ceiling. Slowly lower your hips back down toward the ball and the floor using your arms for support.

C. Repeat for 10 repetitions.

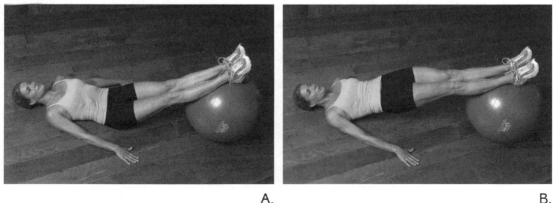

A.   B.

The Leg Circle

Lifting your hips off the floor as you rest your feet on the ball helps create a tighter butt. By working the muscles in your upper legs and alongside your hips, you'll notice better buns in no time!

A. Lie flat on the floor with your lower legs on the ball.

B. Lift your hips and extend your right leg toward the ceiling as you press down into the ball with your left leg. Make five small circles to the right, and then five small circles to the left as you point your toe. Slowly lower your leg back onto the ball and return your hips to the floor.

C. Repeat 5 times for each leg.

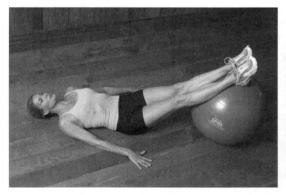
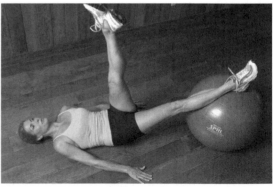

A.   B.

The Tabletop

This exercise is called the "tabletop" because if you keep your hips up and your abdominal muscles pulled in, you will be as flat as a table. Just picture someone having a tea party on your midsection and you'll get the point of this exercise.

A. Sit on the ball with your feet shoulder-width apart. Roll down slowly until only your shoulders and upper back touch the ball. Place your left leg across your right thigh.

B. Lift your hips toward the ceiling as you squeeze or tighten your butt. Hold for a few seconds, then release and lower your hips.

C. Repeat for 5 repetitions before switching legs.

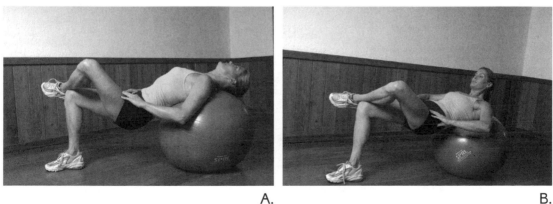

A.   B.

A WORK IN PROGRESS

With so much emphasis on how your body has changed after having a baby, it's comforting to know that so many other women feel the same way, isn't it? In fact, if you've never had the chance to discuss with your own mom or friends how they feel about their body after baby, now would be a good time (most people I know say they still haven't lost their baby fat—and it's fifteen years later).

Accepting yourself just the way you are is the true key to happiness. Challenges will come and go (childbirth being one of the biggest), and each one that you overcome will make you stronger and more determined to get where you're going. Your body may seem different, better in some ways and worse in others, but you're healthy and you're working toward something. Now that's what I call "a work in progress."

6

Six Months After Birth: Sexy Shoulders and Upper Back

How Your Body May Look:
Bloated from a returning period

How You May Be Feeling:
Cramping or anemic from low
iron stores in your body

Equipment Needed:
Resistance band and an exercise ball

"

I am twenty-nine and have had two kids in the last three years. I live in sunny Los Angeles where everyone runs around looking like a model. Here are some of my thoughts about pregnancy and regaining your shape . . . I was twenty-six when I got pregnant with my daughter and gained 40 pounds. I bounced back pretty quickly through occasional exercise and generally being good about what I ate. Within six months, I was back to my pre-pregnancy self. Nine months later, I got pregnant with my son. I had another 40-pound gain but carried very differently. I put on most of the weight in my stomach which, on my 5'1" frame, looked humongous! People often compared my first pregnancy to my second. For me, it was a lose-lose either way!

" I am on my way to losing the weight from my second pregnancy (I'm within 5 pounds of pre-pregnancy weight). Unfortunately, that isn't the hardest part for me. My shape changed and now I'm battling the jelly-belly that looks like I'm still pregnant and a butt-thigh combo that makes me shudder when passing a mirror. I'm even a shoe size bigger! It is very depressing to see okay numbers on the scale but to have a body shape that doesn't resemble my old self is the worst. It feels like I'll never be back in my old clothes! Family and friends try to be supportive and everyone says that it takes time. Of course, we know it takes more than that . . . exercise, diet, and a lot of hard work! "

—Charity Brockman, mother of twenty-month-old Rachel Taylor Brockman, and three-month-old Joshua Alec Brockman

OFFICIAL HALFWAY POINT!

BELIEVE IT OR NOT, it's already been six months since you've had your baby and we are officially at the halfway point! So let's do the math and add up where you are so far in your quest to regain your pre pregnancy shape.

If you gained the recommended 25 to 35 pounds, you will have lost the approximately 12 to 15 pounds from the birth, which left you with around 13 to 20 pounds of weight to be lost when you started this program. Between the walking program in the first two months and the exercises from Chapters 3, 4, and 5, you should be getting much closer to your pre-pregnancy weight in the next couple of months.

Keep in mind, as I mentioned in Chapter 1, you'll need an extra few months for every 5 pounds of weight you gained over 35 pounds. Be patient and remain positive because you will get there!

SIX-MONTH PROGRAM FOR SHOULDERS AND UPPER BACK

At six months you may find yourself in a funk, so to speak, from a returning period. On average, a woman gets her regular period back around this time, and body aches in the shoulders and upper back are quite common. Upper body strength comes into play every time you lift your baby in and out of the crib, in and out of the car seat, in and out the stroller, etc. To help relieve some of the strain you're starting to feel as your baby's getting bigger and harder to carry around, you're going to have to strengthen the muscles in your upper back and to work on toning and defining your shoulders to help you handle the load.

This chapter contains some challenging upper back and shoulder exercises that can be done with a ball and a resistance band. As I mentioned in Chapter 4, "Toned and Shapely Arms and Chest," you'll need a resistance band that is around 5 ½ feet long that you will be able to move easily around the ball to perform the following exercises. Before you begin your workout, start off with a short warm-up consisting of walking, jumping rope, hiking, biking, swimming, or calisthenics. Once you've done that, do all four of the following exercises in this chapter. When you're done with those, try some of the great stretches in Chapter 2 to increase your flexibility.

The Lat Pull

This exercise works to tone and strengthen the lats in the upper back or the area that lies under your bra strap, which can really look bad!

A. Sit on the ball with your feet shoulder-width apart. Begin with your arms up over your head, holding the resistance band in both hands.

B. Bring one arm down to your waist by pulling your elbow toward your rib cage. Raise your arm back above your head and repeat on the other arm.

C. Repeat 10 to 12 repetitions.

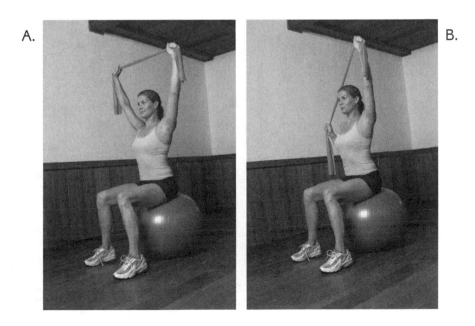

A.

B.

The Upright Row

The upright row exercise is perfect for working your shoulders and upper back. Make sure you sit up tall and maintain your posture when you're on the ball and you'll get a great workout in your tummy!

A. Sit on the ball with your feet shoulder-width apart and place the band under your feet. Your hands will be close to your knees as you hold the resistance band.

B. Slowly pull the band up toward your shoulders as your elbows open out to the sides. Hold for a few seconds before releasing the band and your arms back down to your knees.

C. Repeat 10 to 12 times.

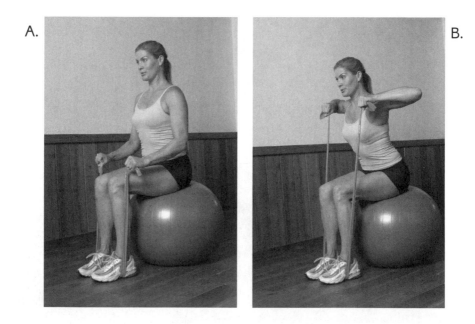

A.   B.

The Rear Delts

This exercise increases strength and works the back of your shoulders, which are usually referred to as your shoulder blades. It also helps tone your arms if you make sure to bring the band back in toward your body slowly after you've finished the pulling move.

A. Sit on the ball with your feet shoulder-width apart. Hold the resistance band in the middle and extend your arms at chest level in front of you.

B. Squeeze your shoulder blades together and pull your arms out to the sides like an airplane. Keeping tension on the band, return your arms to the starting position.

C. Repeat 10 to 12 times.

A.

B.

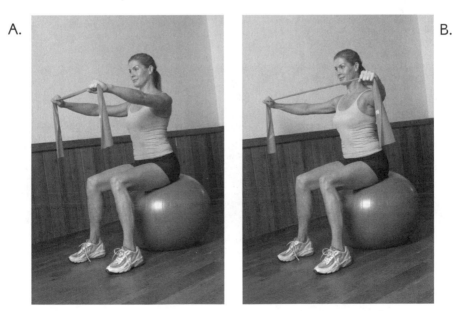

The Fly

Doing fly exercises works to tone the chest and helps lift your breasts. A much-needed exercise for any new mommy!

A. Lie with your upper back and shoulders on the excercise ball and bend your knees at a 90-degree angle. Place the resistance band under your upper back.

B. Extend your arms straight up toward the ceiling directly above your chest so your hands and the resistance band cross at the wrists. Hold for a few seconds before slowly lowering your arms back down to the sides of your body.

C. Repeat 10 to 12 repetitions.

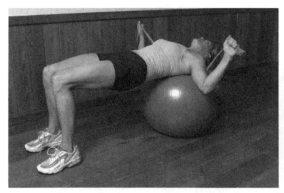
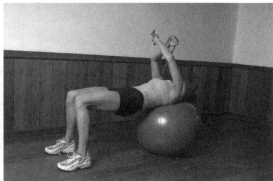

A.   B.

IT ALL ADDS UP

Okay, here's where we talk about eating the baby's food. In case you didn't hear, it's a no-no. And I'm not talking about the stuff that comes in the jar. Oh no, I'm talking about the good stuff—the fish crackers, Cheerios, and those thinly distinguished things they call fruit snacks, etc. Unless you're Kelly Ripa, who says she "lost weight by eating whatever falls off her kid's high chair instead of having four-hour lunches," I really wouldn't recommend it. Most women put on pounds from eating macaroni and cheese and peanut-butter-and-jelly sandwiches—including me (I knew something was wrong when I was hoping my daughter wouldn't finish her taquito).

Eating more of the right things plus eating five to six times throughout the day is important at this stage in the game. To keep you from binging, you need to eat smaller meals of around 300 to 500 calories per meal. A good example would be a piece of fruit and yogurt, or some cottage cheese and crackers. Whatever keeps your energy up and your blood sugar from dipping throughout the day is key. Believe me; it will keep you from looking forward to snacking on Pirate's Booty and pretzels!

7

Seven Months After Birth: Long and Lean Legs

How Your Body May Look:
Approximately 15 inches smaller
or 15 pounds lighter

How You May Be Feeling:
Returning to your old self

Equipment Needed:
A jump rope

How Much Weight You May Have Lost:
A large percentage of women will have dropped
most of their pregnancy weight by now and will
be 15 pounds lighter. However, this doesn't mean
they'll be able to fit into those "skinny jeans" just yet.

66

My first clue that I may have gained a little too much weight during my pregnancy came at my last prenatal visit. It was there that my doctor announced, in front of my husband, that I had gained 65 pounds. Oddly, the look of horror on my husband's face didn't even upset me. I knew that I would be nursing and I thought the weight would just fall off. Imagine my surprise when six months later, I was still carrying around an extra 30 pounds. My stomach looked like Santa Claus—a bowl full of jelly—and any hint of muscle tone in my legs was completely gone. I had no idea that being pregnant and having a baby would change my body so much. I also had no idea how little time and energy I would have to work out and get myself back in shape. **99**

—Kathleen Anne Hunt, mother of two-and-a-half-year-old Cameron

● ● ● ● ● ●
● ○ ○ ○ ○ ○

AS YOU HIT YOUR SEVENTH MONTH post-pregnancy, your body will be somewhere around a total of 15 inches smaller than right after giving birth. That is a combination of bust to waist to hip ratio. Not bad in seven months, huh? Your clothes will be fitting almost as before, but your legs and hips may still be a bit larger—remember, not everything will return to its original size. It is now time to work the legs so we can soon fit into those before-baby clothes.

GETTING ACQUAINTED WITH JUMPING ROPE

Okay, you probably have some childhood memories of jumping or skipping rope that may or may not get you excited about trying it again at this stage in your life. But believe me, whenever I have to be in tip-top shape fast, I grab my jump rope. What else can fit in your bag at a minute's notice and not take up a lot of space? And if any of you have the c-word (cellulite), you may find it interesting to know the only thing that can help (other than liposuction) is jumping rope! By speeding up your circulation, you can flush out all those dents and bumps and look like a boxer in no time. And I do mean *no* time! Jumping rope provides results fast and if you've tried it recently (since you were twelve), you know by now you won't be able to do it very long before feeling like you're ready to quit! So take a moment to read the following list of things you'll need to know to make your transition into becoming a boxer, or just looking like one, a tad smoother.

CROSS TRAINING SHOES OR AEROBIC SHOES: You'll want to make sure you have a pair of cross trainers on hand before you begin jumping rope because they contain extra padding in the ball or front of the foot.

LIGHTWEIGHT JUMP ROPE: You'll want to start off with a jump rope (see Appendix for product information) that doesn't have any kind of added weight to it such as a weighted rope or weighted handles. Both of these devices require extra strength and endurance that should only be used once you become proficient with jumping rope.

WATER . . . LOTS OF IT: You'll want to drink plenty of water and have some extra on hand for the jump-rope program. The more you sweat, the more you should drink, not only to replenish what you've lost but to help flush out the toxins and fatty deposits as your body heats up and begins to sweat.

THE RULES OF JUMPING ROPE

As was the case when you were a kid, there are rules you have to follow to make your experience a successful one when it comes to jumping rope. Here are a few that I think will really help. Good luck!

KEEP YOUR BODY RELAXED AS YOU MAINTAIN A LONG, STRAIGHT BACK: The tendency is to become rigid or stiff as a board when you jump rope, but what you really want to do is remain relaxed so your body can "become one with the rope." The more relaxed you are, the easier it will be for your body to go with the motion, and the better you'll feel after jumping.

USE THE FRONT OF YOUR FEET FOR JUMPING: You'll want to stay light on your feet by using only the front of your foot to jump (otherwise known as the ball of your foot) so you are ready to move each time the rope hits the ground. Keep in mind you are skipping rope and avoid jumping so high that your entire foot comes off the ground. Land on your toes, not on your heels.

DON'T LOOK AT YOUR FEET: You never want to look down at your feet when you're jumping rope unless you want to trip! Be sure to pick a spot on the wall or straight ahead that you can focus on as you're jumping.

KEEP YOUR WRISTS CLOSE TO YOUR BODY: You'll want to keep your wrists and arms close to your body when you're jumping rope so you can maintain control of the movement. Your elbows will also be tucked in close to your body.

JUMP ROPE WORKOUT

So if you have your jump rope and are ready to go, read on to learn the proper way to go about it. But first take the time to do a short warm-up consisting of walking, jogging, jumping jacks, swimming, or biking to get your blood flowing and warm up your muscles properly.

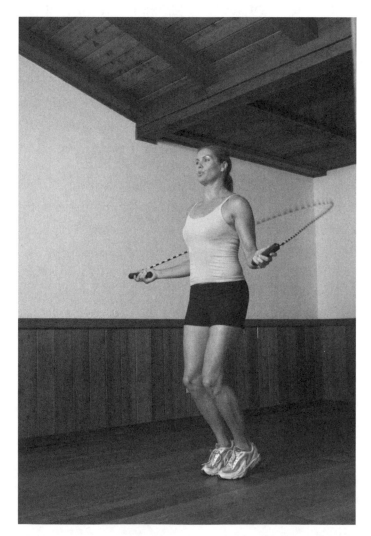

Proper Technique for Jumping Rope

Place both hands at your sides as you hold the handles of your jump rope. Begin by keeping your legs together as you swing the rope over your head and jump. Be sure to use only the balls of your feet to lift off the ground and not your entire foot. Jump as slowly as needed until you feel comfortable enough to speed up while maintaining proper form.

- Because jumping rope is an intense aerobic exercise, you're going to start out slowly with 30-second intervals that contain simple side-to-side movements between each interval for a total workout of 5 minutes.

- Begin by timing your intervals using a sports watch or a kitchen timer.

- Start out jumping rope for 30 seconds or count to 100 (each time the rope hits the ground). When you stop jumping rope, don't stop abruptly to wait for the next 30-second interval. Lunge from side to side or jog in place to keep your body moving at all times.

- Keep jumping rope on and off every 30 seconds, remembering to move in between as you're resting, for a total of five minutes. Try putting on your favorite CD or song that will help to keep the beat of the music as you're skipping rope.

  INCREASING YOUR INTERVALS: When you have mastered the 30-second jump rope intervals as prescribed above, you can increase your jump-roping interval time to 60 seconds or count to 200 each time the rope hits the ground. It may feel like forever but will be worth the amazing results you'll see in your legs and throughout your upper body. By increasing your interval time to one minute and resting for one minute in between, your total workout time will be 10 minutes.

At the end of your jump rope workout, be sure to do a 3- to 5-minute cooldown consisting of lunges from side to side, walking it out, or any exercise that helps your body cool down slowly and allows your breathing to return to normal.

PACKING UP ALREADY?

At seven months, you can start putting some of the toys and clothes away that your baby is outgrowing . . . fast! The bouncy seat and baby bathtub are all things that you may not have use for anymore since your baby is sitting on their own and even crawling around everywhere. Some kids may even try to walk at this point, although my daughter waited until she was one year old (which was perfectly fine with me once I saw how much running I would have to do after her). Whatever the case may be, packing up the 0- to 6-month clothing now is a good idea so it doesn't start piling up as time goes by. And saving only the things that you know you'll reuse is an even smarter idea. I found out the hard way that saving everything Bella had burped up on only resulted in discoloration on her clothes after a few years. Looking back,

I wish I had given some of her "onesies" to my friends who were having babies at the time.

Each stage of having a baby is so wonderful, yet each stage comes with all new types of gadgets and clothing. You'll really be ahead of the game if you clean out the dresser and closet now to make room for the new stuff. And so on, and so on . . .

8

Eight Months After Birth: The Full Body Workout

How Your Body May Look:
Noticeably leaner

How You May Be Feeling:
Energetic and ready to put it all together

Equipment Needed:
Exercise ball and resistance band

66

I'm a first-time mom and I lost the weight very quickly, mostly due to breast-feeding. But, I was still amazed at how much my hips and obviously my breasts had changed. It also seemed like my rib cage had expanded. I am just now, a year later, fitting into some of my pre-pregnancy clothes, even though I lost the weight in about three months. **99**

—Lara Starr, mother of thirteen-month-old Henry Tyler Didden

BELIEVE IT OR NOT, some women find they have a better body after having a baby. For example, women who were athletic before birth may now have a few extra curves and feel more feminine, while others may have actually lost weight and become slimmer. Whatever the case may be, this chapter offers an overall workout that benefits all new moms and incorporates many of the moves from previous chapters. From start to finish, this workout, *consisting of 10 exercises that you perform for 10 repetitions each*, should give you enough time to exercise and still have enough time left over to shower while your baby is napping!

PUTTING IT ALL TOGETHER

The following ball-and-band workout combines many of the toning and strengthening exercises included in this book to make up a great workout that you don't need a huge amount of space for. In addition, there is a warm-up included in this chapter to help to slowly increase your heart rate with some cardio exercises on the ball.

You should start with the warm-up to prepare your body gradually for exercise, then move through the workout at your own pace. In addition, if you really want to get your heart pumping, you can jog in place while holding the ball at chest level, or sit on the ball and do some bouncing. Whatever you choose to do, including a 5- to 10-minute warm-up before every workout is always recommended to avoid injury and to prepare your body for more vigorous exercise.

WARM-UP

The following three exercises provide a warm-up that will prepare you for the next series of exercises. You can use this warm-up with any of the workouts in this book to help increase your circulation and raise your heart rate slowly.

The Side-to-Side Lunge

The side-to-side lunge increases your heart rate as it loosens the muscles in your hamstrings, quads, and butt. Make sure to roll the ball with you for support as you perform each lunge position.

> A. Placing the ball in front of your body within arm's reach, bend to the right side in a lunge position as you touch the ball with your left arm. Place your right arm on your thigh for support.
>
> B. Lunge to the opposite side as you roll the ball along with you.
>
> C. Repeat 10 repetitions to each side.

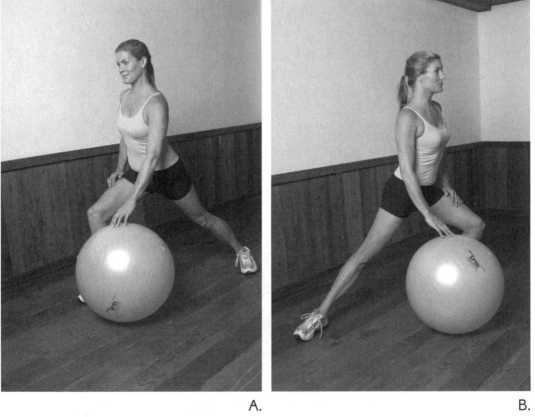

A.   B.

THE BALL REACH

The ball reach combines the squat, which warms up the lower body, with a ball lift to engage the upper body.

A. Holding the ball above your head, stand with your legs straight and your feet a little wider than shoulder-width apart.

B. Bring the ball down toward the floor as you lower your body into a squatting position. Raise the ball back up above your head as you use your heels to press your body up into a standing position.

C. Repeat for 10 repetitions.

A. 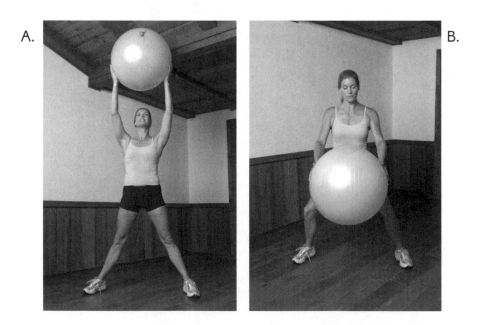 B.

THE BALL SWEEP

Like a pendulum swinging from side to side, you sweep the ball back and forth across your body to perform the ball sweep.

A. Bend your knees in a lunge position as you bring the ball to one side of your body.

B. Bring the ball down toward the floor in a sweeping motion.

C. Continue the sweeping movement with the ball until it reaches the opposite side of your body.

D. Repeat the sweeping motion with the ball to the opposite direction.

E. Repeat for 10 repetitions.

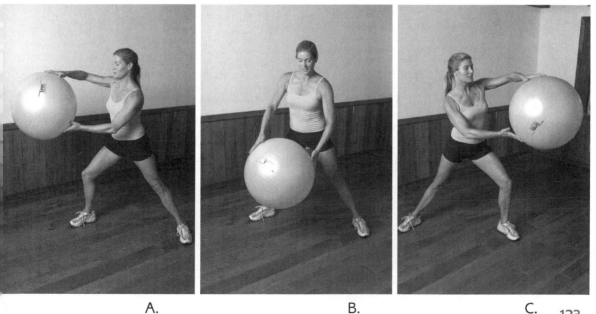

A.   B.   C.

THE UPPER BODY

The next three exercises are pulled from Chapter 4 to provide you with a workout for the upper body. The first two exercises use the resistance band to tone and strengthen while the push-up exercise works the entire chest, shoulders, arms, and upper back.

The Overhead Press

With the help of a resistance band, the overhead press works the arms and shoulders to make lifting all that baby stuff a little easier.

> A. Sit on the ball with your feet shoulder-width apart and place the band securely under your feet. Hold the ends of the band in your hands at shoulder level, being sure to keep your palms facing forward.
>
> B. Straighten your arms above your head and hold for a few seconds. Slowly bring your arms back to shoulder level or starting position.
>
> C. Repeat 10 to 12 repetitions.

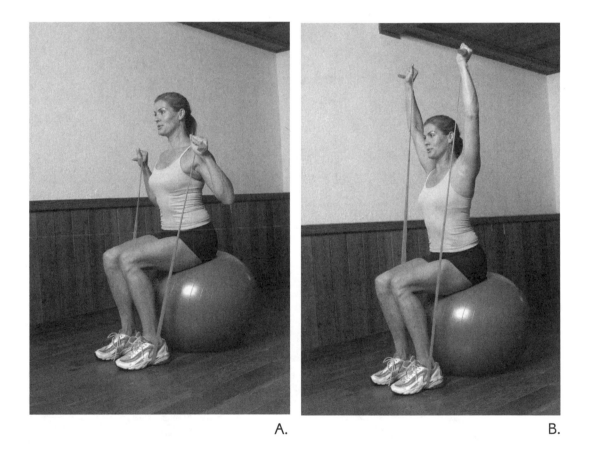

A.   B.

The Chest Press

The chest press helps to lift and tone the breasts by building and strengthening the pectoral muscles.

A. Lie with your upper back and shoulders on the ball. Place the resistance band under your upper back and the ball as you hold the ends of the band in each hand. Your thighs should be parallel to the floor.

B. With your elbows bent to the sides, press your arms to the ceiling as you contract the muscles in your chest and tighten your stomach muscles. Return to the starting position by relaxing your elbows back to your body and even with your shoulders.

C. Repeat 10 times.

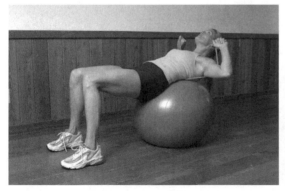
A.

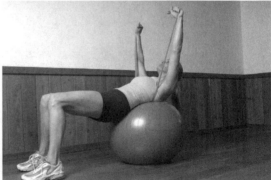
B.

The Push-Up

There's nothing better than a push-up for working your upper body. When combined with the ball, this exercise helps strengthen your core as you pull in your abdominal muscles and maintain a long, straight back.

A. Lie with your belly on the ball and walk your hands forward until the ball rests under your lower legs or shins. Make sure that you keep your hands directly below your shoulders.

B. Lower your upper body toward the floor, bending the elbows out to the sides. Straighten the elbows and exhale as you press back up into starting position.

C. Repeat 10 times.

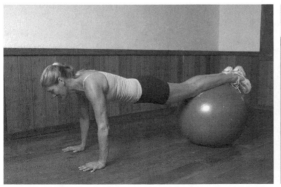
A.

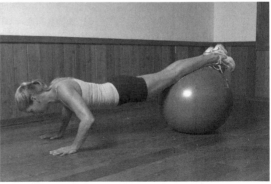
B.

THE LOWER BODY

The next series of exercises are pulled from Chapter 5 to provide a lower body workout. These exercises will help strengthen and tone your lower body by using the ball and gravity for resistance.

The Hip Lift

This exercise requires you to use the strength of your hips and butt to lift your body weight off the floor.

A. Lie flat on the floor with your feet and ankles on top of the ball. Your arms will be alongside your body on the floor for support.

B. Pressing down into the ball with your feet to maintain your balance, exhale as you raise your hips and pelvis toward the ceiling. Slowly lower your hips back down toward the ball and the floor using your arms for support.

C. Repeat for 10 repetitions.

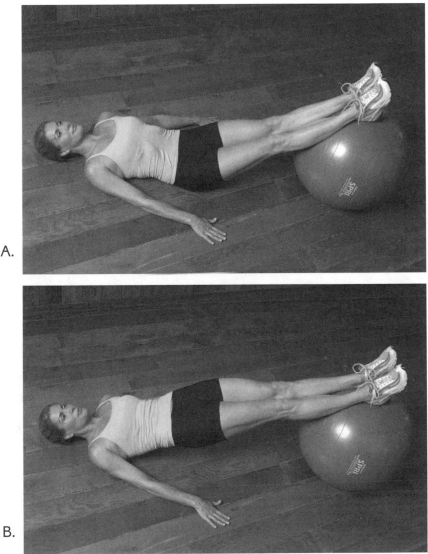

A.

B.

The Leg Circle

This is a great exercise for lengthening and strengthening your legs. It also works the hips and glutes as you press your body weight into the ball to keep it steady.

A. Lie flat on the floor with your lower legs on the ball.

B. Lift your hips and extend your right leg toward the ceiling as you press down into the ball with your left leg. Make five small circles to the right, and then five small circles to the left as you point your toe. Slowly lower your leg back onto the ball and return your hips to the floor.

C. Repeat 5 times for each leg.

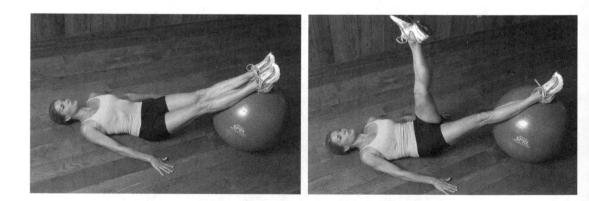

THE FINAL STRETCH

The following exercises are pulled from Chapter 2 to help you stretch out at the end of your workout. You can use these stretching exercises after completing any of the workouts in this book to help increase your flexibility and release any tightness in your muscles.

The Quads Stretch

This stretch helps relieve tightness in the muscle that lies in front of your thigh, otherwise known as your quadriceps.

A. Lie with your tummy on the ball so it is directly under your hips. To maintain your balance, place your right hand and right leg on the floor as you lift your left leg behind you. Raise your left arm and reach behind you to grab your left ankle. Stretch the front of your leg using a gentle pulling motion. Lower your left arm and left leg to the floor before repeating on the other side.

B. Repeat 3 times on each leg.

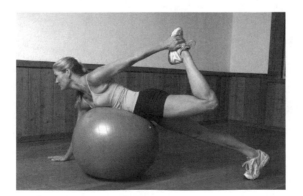

The Drape

The drape is the most effective of all the stretching exercises to stretch out your spine and lower back. This exercise is a great way to end any workout on the ball. For an easier variation, see page 60.

A. Place your tummy on the ball and drape your entire body over the ball.

B. Once you feel comfortable, rest your fingertips on the floor in front of you for an extra stretch. Return to starting position and rest on your knees before repeating.

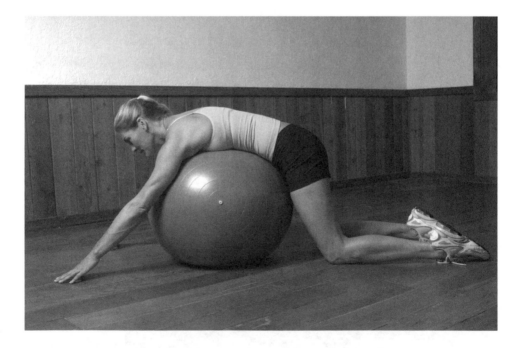

STOPPING TO SMELL THE ROSES

Getting started on any new exercise program is tough, but once you get into doing it regularly, it becomes easier and easier. Then, just when you feel you're reaching the point of knowing it so well you could do it in your sleep, it becomes time to take a break and evaluate the progress you've made so far.

The same thing can be said for the time you spend trying to be a good mother—you probably never stop and take a look at the small accomplishments you've made up to this point. And if you don't, before you know it your baby will have entered an entirely new stage that comes with a whole new set of problems to solve. So enjoy watching *The Wiggles* three times in a row, or reading your baby a story over and over that you think she doesn't seem to be listening to, because before you know it, your baby will start talking and telling you some amazing things that will surprise even Mommy.

9

Nine Months After Birth: Circuit Training Program

How Your Body May Look:
Pre-pregnancy weight

How You May Be Feeling:
Ready to try on those skinny jeans!

Equipment Needed:
Jump rope and a coffee table

"

I gained between 35 and 40 pounds with my son. I've always been relatively thin but if I ever gained any weight it was always in the belly . . . I never had a six-pack! So I loved being pregnant and not having to suck in my stomach. Fortunately, I didn't have swelling ankles or anything like that, but after giving birth I definitely had the post-pregnancy pooch. I remember my friend came over when the baby was about five days old and said, "It's so good to see Heather fat for once in her life." (I tried to remind myself that this is the same friend who said to me on my wedding day, "Remind me never to get married in the Valley; it's way too freaking hot here.") Anyway, I set out to lose the pooch by eating less and eating right and because I live in the San Fernando Valley (which, contrary to my friend's belief, is not always hot) I found I was able to take two to three walks a day, because my son Drake would fall asleep on the walks and I'd come home and be able to make myself a salad. That's when I saw **Oprah** and she said to stop eating three hours before you go to bed because when you feel those little hunger pains, that means your body is feeding off your fat and you'll lose weight. That helped a bit but in reality, it took close to nine months to finally be able to fit back into every piece of clothing I had and still I wish I would have worked on my stomach because it just doesn't look the same. **"**

—Heather McDonald Tobias, mother to two-year-old Drake, step-mom to five-year-old Mackenzie, and expecting baby number two

● ● ● ● ● ●
● ● ● ○ ○ ○

NINE MONTHS UP, NINE MONTHS DOWN! Maybe you are where you were when you started this journey, and maybe you're not. Try on those skinny jeans . . . you may just be surprised. Nine months after I had Bella, boredom set in and I knew I needed to switch my fitness routine, and I'll bet you're feeling the same right about now. Whether it's walking, hiking, biking, spinning, yoga, pilates, tap dancing, hip hop, or kickboxing, exercising a new muscle group can provide fast results and beat boredom. Because your body can get "stuck" at a certain weight sometimes, adding something new to your exercise program can give you the results you're looking for. Circuit training, where you work a body part intensely for short intervals with only 30 seconds of rest in between before switching to another body part, is a new and fun way to work out. By constantly changing the muscle group you are exercising, you can burn more calories and shock your body into a new zone to get better results.

This chapter contains a circuit-training program that I designed for new moms to help them get results fast. You can do it anywhere, anytime, and all you need is one simple piece of equipment—a coffee table. Yes, that's right—a coffee table. And you can even use this workout when you travel because all you have to do is clear a small space in your hotel room and voilà; you instantly have a mini gym (now you never have the excuse not to work out, darn). The following circuit workout is simple, fast, and fun, plus I've added the jump-rope routine from Chapter 7 to burn some extra calories. So let's get started!

COFFEE TABLE WORKOUT

Grab your coffee table, jump rope, and a towel because you are going to give Hillary Swank a run for her money with your very own boxer's workout to whip your butt into shape—fast! And don't forget your water because you'll need to re-hydrate from all the sweating you'll be doing . . .

SETTING UP YOUR CIRCUIT: To set up your circuit-training area, you'll need enough space to jump rope and have your coffee table off to one side. If you don't have enough room to jump rope in the area where your coffee table is, you can perform jumping jacks or jump without the rope. You'll also want to leave yourself enough room to walk back and forth and lunge from one side of the room to the other. Let's begin!

Interval 1: Jump Rope

To provide a total body warm-up and burn lots of calories, you'll start your circuit with the jump rope routine from Chapter 7.

A. Begin with 100 counts or 30 seconds of jumping rope. You can do this by counting every time the rope hits the floor. When you get to 100 counts, drop your rope.

Keep moving for 30 seconds or as you count to 100.

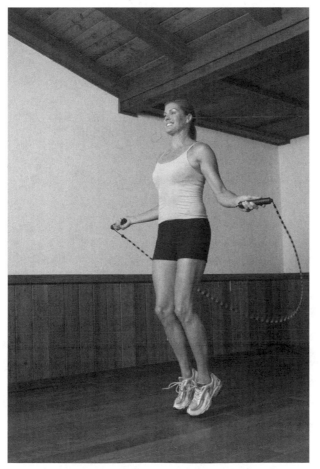

Interval 2: Lunges

For the second exercise in your circuit, you'll be doing lunges from one side of the room to the other. Lunges are a good way to tone and strengthen your thighs and butt.

A. Take a big step forward with your right leg and bend your right knee as you lower down into lunge position. Take a big step forward with your left leg and sink down into a lunge position with your left knee.

B. Perform 5 lunges to the opposite side of the room. Turn around and do 5 lunges back to the other side of the room. You will finish exactly where you started. Keep moving for thirty seconds or as you count to 100.

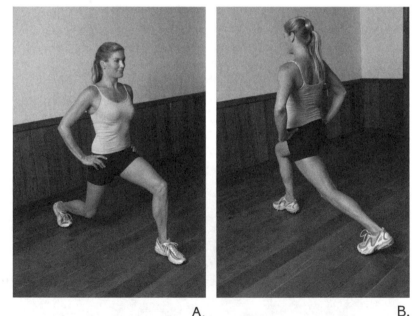

A.   B.

Interval 3: Push-Ups

A coffee table push-up will be next in line for your circuit workout. This excersise works the chest, arms, shoulders, and upper back.

A. Standing and facing your coffee table, place your hands on the edge of the table for support as you straighten your arms and extend your legs back behind you.

B. Inhale as you lower your chest to the table in a classic push-up position by bending your elbows out to the side. Exhale as you press back up to your starting position. Make sure you keep your back flat. (As you become more advanced, you can place the tops of your feet on the coffee table and perform push-ups off the floor).

C. Perform 10 push-ups.
Keep moving for thirty seconds or as you count to 100.

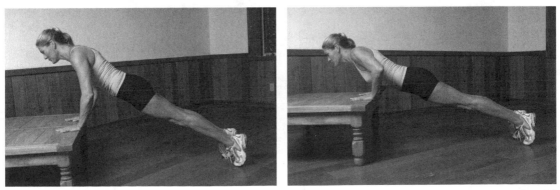

A.   B.   141

Interval 4: Sit-ups

The next exercise in your circuit is a coffee table sit-up. Instead of doing regular sit-ups with your feet flat on the floor, you will be resting your feet on the coffee table, which really helps to flatten your tummy.

A. Lie on your back with your knees bent and your heels on the coffee table.

B. Place your hands behind your head with your elbows out to the sides and lift your shoulders off the floor toward the ceiling.

C. Perform 10 sit-ups.

D. Keep moving for thirty seconds or as you count to 100.

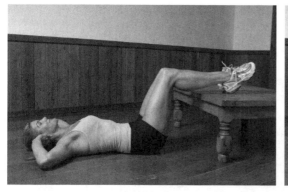
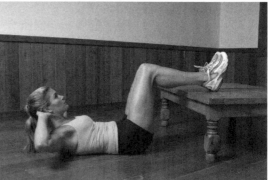

A.   B.

Interval 5: Squats

For the fifth exercise in your circuit, you will be doing squats that work all the large muscle groups in the lower half of your body.

A. With your arms out in front of you at chest level, lower down in a squatting position so your knees are parallel to the floor or as far as you can go. Exhale as you press back up into a standing position.

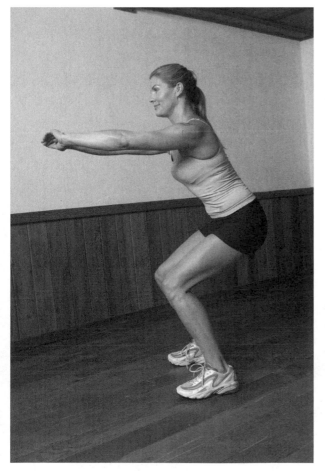

B. Perform 10 squats fast.

C. Keep moving for thirty seconds or as you count to 100.

Interval 6: Dips

For the final exercise in your circuit, you will be performing dips to work the muscles along the backs of your arms called triceps.

A. With your back facing the coffee table, bend your knees and place your hands behind you on the table. Cross one leg on top of the opposite knee.

B. Inhale as you bend your elbows and lower or dip your body down toward the floor. Exhale as you straighten your arms and press back up.

C. Perform 10 dips.

D. Keep moving for thirty seconds or as you count to 100. **Repeat circuit one more time.**

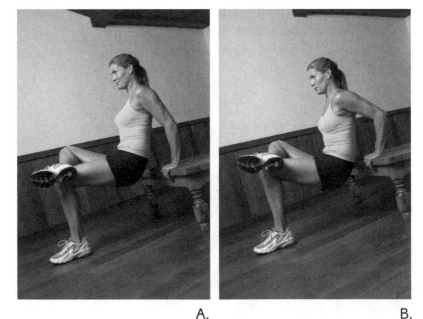

A.   B.

WALKING AND TALKING

Walking is such a great exercise because you don't need anything but your feet to get you where you're going. Plus, you can bring your baby along! And not only does it provide fresh air and exercise as I mentioned in Chapter 2, but it gives you a chance to meet other moms like yourself in your own neighborhood. It seems like every time I go outside, I see a mom pushing a stroller or carrying a baby in a sling and I didn't even know there were other moms who lived around me. And many times when I'm out pushing Bella in her jogging stroller, my neighbors give me shouts of encouragement. I remember one lady saying, "You're looking great! Keep it up." Those few simple words of encouragement helped me to keep going when I really didn't feel like it at all sometimes.

So stick with walking no matter what stage you and your baby happen to be in. Those words of encouragement may come from your very own next-door neighbor just when you need them most!

10

Ten Months After Birth: Weight Training Program

How Your Body May Look:
You may have lost a total of 40 pounds

How You May Be Feeling:
Hormonally back to normal

Equipment Needed:
10- to 15-pound dumbbells and an exercise ball

66

I only gained 23 pounds when I was pregnant. My weight gain was low because I delivered my daughter early due to health problems. About a month after I gave birth, my daughter had an appointment with a gastroentrologist (for digestive disorders). At that appointment, I spotted a scale and weighed myself. I was shocked to see that I was down to 123 pounds. I was about 125 pounds when I first became pregnant. I was still wearing maternity clothes because I hadn't realized that the weight was gone. My husband would tell me that I looked skinny, but I thought he was just humoring me! I tried on my blue jeans when I arrived home and was shocked to see that they fit.

66 Unfortunately, the GI specialist. found that my daughter was unable to digest proteins, and was having a hard time with my breast milk and the foods I ate. So I was put on a strict diet where I couldn't eat foods containing dairy, soy, eggs, fish, shellfish, nuts, or peanuts. By the time my daughter was four and a half months old, I was down to 109 pounds. I finally had to throw in the towel with breast-feeding and put my daughter on hypoallergenic formula. I never thought having a baby would make me skinny! Who knew? Since then I've put my weight back on and am back to 120 pounds. I feel so much healthier! **99**

—Cheryl Dorfman, mother of seventeen-month-old
Amy Dorfman

NOT EVERYBODY HAS A PROBLEM LOSING WEIGHT after having a baby, but *everybody* has a difficult time looking the way they would like to. Being healthy and feeling good about yourself is really what it's all about, isn't it? And at a rate of 4 pounds a month, which is very safe and realistic, you may now have shed around 40 pounds making your body ready to tone, tone, and tone. Because muscle burns a lot more calories than fat does, now is a good time to switch to strength training using weights to tone and trim your body.

In this chapter, you will use heavier dumbbells with the following exercises to enable your body to increase muscle mass and burn more fat. If you normally use 3- to 5-pound weights, you will need to increase that amount to 10 to 15 pounds or an amount of weight that allows you to do no more than 10 to 12 repetitions. By using heavier weights, you will build muscle and increase your metabolism, which results in losing fat. Plus, the more muscle you have, the more calories you will burn throughout the day and the night—as the saying goes, "Burn calories while you sleep."

WEIGHT TRAINING GUIDELINES

When you are just beginning to use weights, there are a few guidelines you should follow. Read on to find out more about what you need to know before weight training.

149

1. Warm up properly to avoid injury by doing a light set of each exercise using lighter weights or doing cardio such as jumping jacks, jumping rope, or walking.

2. Pick an amount of weight that only allows you to do 10 to 12 repetitions.

3. Don't forget to breathe or exhale with effort as you lift the weights and inhale as you release the weights.

4. Slowly release the weights when you are finished with each exercise.

5. Start with only one set of each exercise. As you grow stronger, add on another set.

6. When you have reached two sets of each exercise, start adding on *one* repetition. Never exceed 15 repetitions.

7. Work a new muscle group every day—don't use the same muscle group two days in a row.

8. To see the most improvement, have a day of rest in-between weight training sessions.

WEIGHT TRAINING PROGRAM ON THE BALL

The exercises in this chapter combine 10- to 15-pound weights with the exercise ball for a powerful and fun workout. Make sure you have enough space to move your ball around because you will be sitting, lying, and standing up against the wall for the following weight training program.

The Biceps Curl

In this exercise, using the ball to engage your core muscles as you work on your biceps gives you more bang for your buck!

A. Sit on the ball with your feet hip-width apart and your weights down by your sides.

B. Slowly curl your weights toward your shoulders, yours palms facing toward you, as you pull in your abdominal muscles. Hold for a few seconds before releasing the weights back down to your sides.

C. Complete one set of 10 to 12 repetitions.

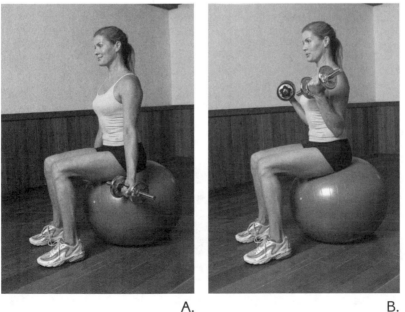

A.   B.

The Shoulder Press

You'll be working the shoulders in this exercise and engaging your core to stay seated on the ball.

A. Sit on the ball with your feet hip-width apart. Bring your weights to shoulder level with your palms facing front.

B. Exhale as you press the weights upward towards the ceiling. Make sure your arms are fully extended at the top. Inhale as you slowly bring your arms back down into the starting position.

C. Complete one set of 10 to 12 repetitions.

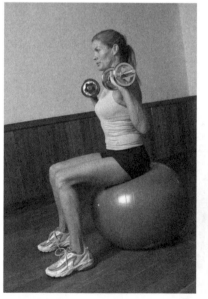
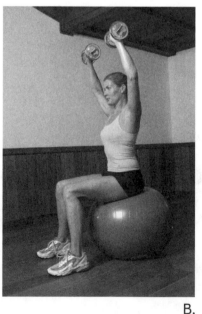

A. B.

The Lateral Arm Raise

This exercise is perfect to work the top of your shoulders and help lose the bulge under your bra strap.

A. Sit on the ball with your feet hip-width apart and bring your weights to your waist. Your palms will be facing in toward your body.

B. Keeping your hands and weights even with your elbows, raise your arms out sideways, stopping at shoulder level. Tighten your abdominal muscles as you bring your arms back down to the starting position.

C. Complete one set of 10 to 12 repetitions.

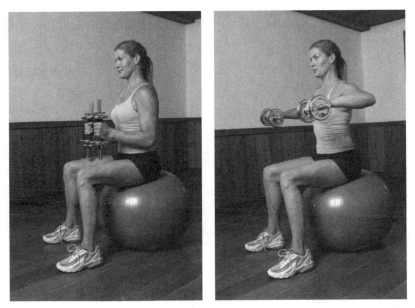

A.   B.

153

The Triceps Press

To work the back of your arms and keep them from getting flabby, this is my favorite exercise.

A. Sit on the ball with your feet hip-width apart and hold one weight in both hands behind your head. Your elbows will be close to your forehead.

B. Pressing the weight toward the ceiling, straighten your elbows behind your head. Slowly lower the weight back down behind your neck.

C. Complete one set of 10 to 12 repetitions.

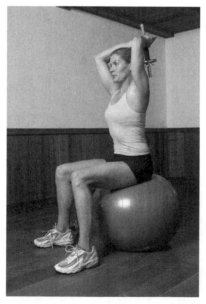

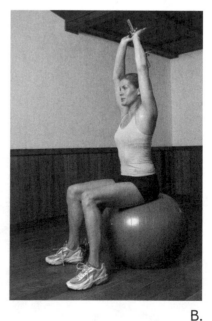

A.   B.

The Upright Rows

It takes a lot of effort to keep the ball steady during this exercise. As a result, this exercise works both your upper and lower body very nicely.

A. Place your right knee on the ball and balance yourself by placing your right hand next to it. Your left leg will be on the floor for support.

B. Holding the weight in your left hand at your side, pull the weight up with a rowing motion as your elbow pulls back past your rib cage. Hold for a few seconds then release the weight down to your side.

C. Complete 10 repetitions, then switch sides and repeat.

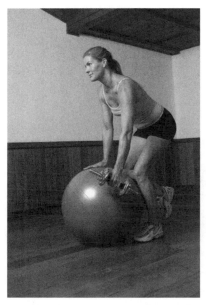 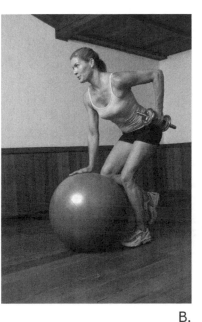

A.   B.

The Bicep Curls with a Wall Squat

To combine upper-body strengthening with lower-body toning, the biceps curl with a wall squat does it all.

A. With the weights in your hands, position the ball behind your back.

B. Slowly squat down as the ball rolls along the wall, as you bring the weights in toward your shoulders to perform a biceps curl. Slowly release the weights back down to your sides and straighten your knees to return to starting positon.

C. Complete 10 repetitions.

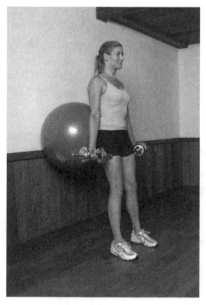

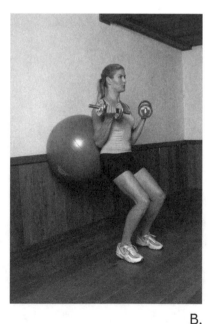

A.   B.

The Bridge with Chest Press

This exercise works the pectoral muscles to give your breasts a lift along with working your hips, butt, and hamstrings.

A. With a weight in each hand, rest your upper back and shoulders on the ball making sure your knees are bent at a 90-degree angle. Be sure to keep your hips lifted.

B. Extend your arms directly above your chest pushing your weights toward the ceiling. Your palms will be facing forward as you press your weights up. Slowly lower your weights by bending your elbows in toward your body.

C. Complete one set of 10 repetitions.

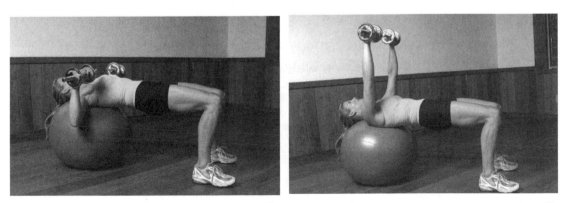

A.   B.

ALL OR NOTHING?!

Having an all-or-nothing approach to fitness is pretty much considered "old school" nowadays. The same can be said for telling people the truth about your age (but that's an entirely different subject that even I don't like to talk about). Yes, gone are the days when you have to have a full 60 minutes to work out—and all you have to do is change your thinking and start using the time you do have to get fit instead of worrying about the time you don't have.

I was just telling someone about my program the other day and they said, "Can you really get a workout in 10 minutes?" Well, as you know by now if you've read this book the answer is yes! You can get a work out in 10 minutes and you can get a great one. Plus, you can do it twice a day and now you're already at 20 minutes! Just like starting and stopping a video that you use to work out at home, you can do the same with your at-home workouts. And because you don't have to leave the house, you don't have the travel time back and forth to the gym, which is even better.

So get out there and walk, bike, jump rope (my personal favorite), swim or jog in place and do some push-ups, because it all adds up and it's a fact—it's better than doing nothing!

11

Eleven Months After Birth: Running After Your Baby!

How Your Body May Look: Strong

How You May Be Feeling: Exhausted

Equipment Needed: A jogging stroller

"

I am a first-time mom and would be really interested in some tips on using a jogging stroller. Is it best to jog with two hands or alternate left and right? Should you extend your arms on a hill or relax them? I always end up hunched over the stroller and have to remind myself to straighten my back. I worry that I will strain a muscle or hurt my back due to incorrect form. I was just thinking about this today and was hoping you could provide me with the answers. **"**

—Lara Starr, mother of thirteen-month-old Henry
Tyler Didden

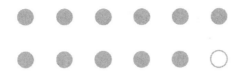

RIGHT AROUND ONE YEAR, your "crawler" will start walking and you will need all the help you can get! Keeping on your toes, so to speak, will make all the difference in the world when it's time to not only chase but also keep up with your baby. Now is the time to invest in a three-wheeled jogger so Baby can get used to sitting in it while you go, go, go. It's a great way for your curious little boy or girl to see the world and it will help to keep you in tip-top shape. Remember, energy begets energy. This chapter contains a running or jogging program that can be used well into the second year or whenever your toddler stops wanting to sit! But first, let's take a look at what a jogging stroller actually is and which one is right for you.

WHAT EXACTLY IS A JOGGING STROLLER?

A jogging stroller is different from a baby stroller because it has three wheels instead of four and is made specifically for handling faster movements and making quicker turns. Most doctors don't recommend using jogging strollers for babies until they are at least six months old and can hold their heads up on their own. I personally think right around a year is the best time to begin using a jogging stroller because of the possible bumping and jarring that can take place when you're running or jogging (although your baby will find this amusing—trust me).

Jogging strollers come in all different sizes and shapes with the wheel size being the thing that differentiates one jogging stroller from another. And the wheel size you pick largely depends on what kind of workout you will be doing and where, because the larger the wheels, the more comfort the jogging stroller provides. For example, a heavy-duty jogging stroller that you use with rocky terrain has wheels that are 20 inches or larger, whereas a lightweight jogging stroller has 16-inch wheels.

Prices for jogging strollers range anywhere from $99 to $200 or even higher in some instances. Whatever price range you chose, make sure your jogging stroller has deep seats for your child to sit in for added protection and safety straps to be strapped in tight. It's also a good idea to invest in a helmet for your little one just to be extra safe and get him or her in the habit of wearing one early. And last but not least, pick a route with your child in mind that doesn't have too many bumps and jags.

PROPER FORM FOR USING A JOGGING STROLLER

Maintaining proper form is more difficult than you'd think when using a jogging stroller because the extra weight and resistance your baby adds to your workout can place strain on your lower back. The tendency is to lean forward or bend at the waist to push your stroller instead of maintaining a straight back with your abdominal muscles pulled in tight. The bottom line—if you keep your abdominal muscles pulled in while you're pushing your stroller, you'll protect your back and be able to maintain proper form. To help strengthen your core or midsection, see the exercises in Chapter 3.

When it comes to the handles of your stroller, make sure the handles are right around waist level so you can push the stroller comfortably without leaning forward. You don't want the handles to be too low because it will cause you to start bending forward at the waist to push instead of maintaining a straight back. You'll also want to keep your elbows bent and into your body and not straightened out in front of you.

A FEW MORE TIPS FOR USING PROPER FORM WITH YOUR JOGGING STROLLER:

- Keep your back straight and lead with your chest.

- Take long strides with your toes facing forward.

- Keep your wrists straight as you maintain a slight bend in your arms.

- Always keep both hands on your stroller because it is made to roll along with you and can easily get away from you.

- Keep your shoulders pulled back and not hunched forward or let them rise up toward your ears.

163

JOGGING STROLLER WORKOUT

The best thing about using a jogging stroller as opposed to a regular stroller is that you can take it so many fun places. You can go to the beach and go roller blading or take it hiking and push it down a nature trail.

The following jogging stroller workout can be done anywhere you find flat terrain and a small hill in the same vicinity because you will be doing some light jogging and pushing your stroller up a hill. Because the total time for this workout is around 30 minutes and includes the baby, you will have to fit it in-between naps (unless your baby likes to sleep in the stroller like mine does) or pick a time of day that best suits you and your baby's schedule.

- Pick a destination that you can easily repeat daily.

- Start off with fifteen jumping jacks.

- Jog in place to the count of 100.

- Start out walking using a moderate pace on flat terrain for 5 minutes.

- Walk up a small hill and back down using a slower pace. Repeat two more times.

- Continue walking on flat terrain at a fast pace for 5 minutes.

- Stop and face your jogging stroller. Holding on to the handles of your stroller, perform squats exercises (see Chapter 9 for illustration) for 1 minute.

- Jog lightly on flat terrain for 5 minutes.

- Finish walking on flat terrain at a slow pace for 5 to 10 minutes.

LEADING BY EXAMPLE?

It occurred to me the other day, just how much kids copy what you do and say. Yikes! Like all parents, I try to set a good example and make the best choices for my family. But it's the little things like swimming along with your kids in the pool or running back and forth on the sidelines at their soccer game that really sends them the message that you like to be active. Not only does being active set up your kids for living a healthier lifestyle, but it also helps them adopt a good attitude about exercise for the rest of their lives. So next time you're at the park, go ahead and play on the monkey bars, bring your jump rope along, or go down the slide, because you never know who's watching . . .

12

Twelve Months After Birth: Anybody Want Another Baby?

How Your Body May Look:
Back to your pre-pregnancy shape,
if not better!

How You May Be Feeling:
Somewhat melancholy

Equipment Needed:
Baby photo album, to remember what
your little bundle of joy first looked like

"

Our first son, Travis, was conceived through IVF (after three tries and $25,000) so becoming pregnant with our second baby when Travis was only twelve months old was a complete shock. When I got pregnant, he was still a 'baby' in my eyes. How on earth was I going to take care of two babies? It was a blessing, but we were scared.

" However, by the time Owen was born, Travis was twenty months old and had grown up so much. I now think the age difference between them is perfect, and I'm glad to get all the difficult years (diapers, no sleep, etc.) out of the way at once. Plus, I know that in a couple more years, they'll be buddies and will be able to entertain themselves, so Mommy will finally get a break! **"**

—Erin Newman, mother of five-month-old Owen and two-year-old Travis

● ● ● ● ● ●

● ● ● ● ● ●

OH, THE MEMORIES. Seems like just yesterday you were holding your little bundle of joy in the hospital. But it's been a year and quite possibly you're feeling like it's time to have another one, although doctors say it's best to wait eighteen months after having a baby before becoming pregnant again. And to that I say—it's hard enough planning ahead for a dental visit these days let alone planning ahead for a baby!

In this chapter, I address how to take the exercises in this book and continue them throughout the twelfth month and beyond to keep you looking fit and feeling good. And later on in this chapter, you'll find questions from other moms who share common concerns about their bodies beyond the one-year mark.

KEEPING OFF THE WEIGHT

When I was doing research for this book, I came across some pretty staggering statistics about women and weight loss. One of the most interesting things I read really stuck in my mind because it pretty much applies to every woman I know whether they've had a baby or not—if you gain only 2 pounds each year, you will be 20 pounds heavier in ten years (so that explains why so many women come up to me and say, "I had my baby fifteen years ago and I still haven't lost my baby fat!"). The fact is weight gain doesn't happen overnight at all—it creeps up

169

on you gradually. And as you grow older and your metabolism slows down, it becomes harder and harder to maintain your "high school figure"—no matter who you are.

If you do decide to have another baby you will have to work twice as hard to get your shape back and I know plenty of women who have multiple kids who look absolutely fabulous. However, once you have a baby it becomes much harder to maintain your shape because of all the changes your body went through when you were pregnant and gave birth. Your hips may have been stretched out or your abdominal muscles may have slackened from being pregnant and, of course, your breasts may not look the same (be sure to read "I Hate the Way My Boobs Look" at the end of this chapter).

So to keep yourself looking and feeling your best no matter how many babies you have, read on to find the best workouts you can use from this book to achieve your goal.

COMPONENTS TO KEEPING YOUR NEW FIT BODY

Here is a list of the best workouts in this book you can do to maintain your shape now and for as long as you desire.

> TEN MINUTES, TWICE-A-DAY: The number one thing you can do to keep the weight off and stay trim is by incorporating the 10-minute twice-a-day workouts in this book into your everyday life. Doing shorter 10-minute workouts is realistic and cumulative—meaning it all adds up. It also helps boost your metabolism by

getting your heart rate up twice a day to burn calories more efficiently. And the best thing it does is to *not* let you use the excuse that you don't have enough time, because everybody has 10 minutes.

WALKING AND STROLLER PROGRAM: Walking is the number one form of exercise I recommend for every stage in your life—before becoming pregnant, while you are pregnant, and right after having a baby. In Chapters 2 and 11 of this book, I lay out a program that can easily be done with your baby when they're either small enough to use a stroller or big enough to sit by themselves in a jogging stroller (and if you have two kids or twins, there are double joggers). Both of these exercise programs use the weight and resistance of your baby to help you achieve amazing results.

JUMP ROPE PROGRAM: Jumping rope is something you can do to maintain your new shape whether you're traveling, the kids are napping, or you just don't have a lot of time for working out. In Chapter 7, I provide a jump rope program that takes minimal time and provides maximum results in only 5 minutes! Plus, jumping rope is an all-over body toning exercise that provides a killer cardiovascular workout and can incinerate calories and get rid of cellulite at the same time. Yay!

1,400 CALORIE EATING PLAN: The eating plan in this chapter was designed to help you eat more of the right things and less of the sugary, fatty foods that will cause you to gain weight. The well-balanced, easy-to-follow eating plan included here also follows the principle I mentioned in Chapter 1 of eating five to six times a day rather than eating three full meals, which only leads to a drop in blood sugar and low energy levels.

COMMON CONCERNS FOR WOMEN BEYOND THE ONE-YEAR MARK

Whether it's stretch marks, a pooch tummy, hair loss, or breast-feeding issues after a year, every mom wonders if she'll ever look and feel the same as she did before she gave birth. The following letters share some of the most common concerns women have and how to counter them with natural remedies and, well, lots of hard work!

" I Didn't Regain My Shape After Each Baby . . . "

"My husband and I had a plan: we would have two kids right away after we got married and then see about the third. After having my first, I relaxed for nine months and didn't worry about losing the baby weight; I just wanted to enjoy my baby. Then I decided to eat right and exercise so I loaded my baby into a jogging stroller and walked away the fat, five days a week for 50 minutes. Three months later (and one year after my first baby was born), I was 10 pounds away from my goal and pregnant with my second. After my second was born, I relaxed for six months, then loaded the two kids into a double jogging stroller and walked five days a week for 50 minutes. After three months of walking (and nine months after my second baby was born), I was 7 pounds away from goal and surprise, baby number three was on the way!

Now I have three little ones ages 3 ½, 1 ½ and 4 months. I want to lose the baby fat! I am now 19 pounds away from my goal and I really wish I would have known how important it was to be back to my original weight before getting pregnant! I feel like I don't even know my body anymore. I was twenty-eight when I started my baby-making machine and now I am almost thirty-three. I feel like I lost time and I can't go back! I am tired of wearing fat clothes and want to be able to wear all of the latest fashions with confidence. I am going to have to finally get on an exercise plan and stop eating like I am still eating for two. I believe I can do it! I want to be able to wear a bikini and look good in it. I want people to say to me, 'Wow, you look great.'"

—Janay Schrier, mother of three-and-a-half-year-old Justin, one-year-old Jenna, and four-month-old Jewel

Janay is a good example of someone who tried to get back to her pre-pregnancy weight before having more kids but unfortunately waited too long to begin exercising after each birth. If you've read this book, you know by now that it's important to start early, no matter how difficult it may seem. And if you are preparing for baby number two or three, it's time to get started. Getting a jumpstart on regaining your shape before you go for the next baby definitely makes it easier in the long run to get your figure back.

The good news is Janay is only 19 pounds away from her pre-pregnancy weight. Simply by modifying the way she eats, using portion control, and adding a few more days to her regular walking routine, Janay will be able to get the results she's looking for. And because her metabolism is still good at her age of thirty-three, she has a great chance of dropping the weight quickly and still have enough energy to chase all three of her kids around the house with an easy-to-follow 1,400-calorie-a-day eating plan.

1,400 CALORIE EATING PLAN

The following is a sample menu that lists each food and the number of calories it contains next to it so you can exchange one food group for another if you like.

Breakfast:

1 egg (75 calories)

1 slice whole-wheat toast (100 calories)

Mid-morning:

1 ounce of cheese (100 calories)

1 apple (90 calories)

Lunch:

>4 ounces skinless chicken breast (150 calories)

>½ cup cooked veggies (50 calories)

>1 cup green salad (100 calories)

Mid-Afternoon:

>1 cup fruit / cantaloupe (60 calories)

Dinner:

>4 ounces of salmon (175 calories)

>¾ cups pasta (200 calories)

>½ cup cooked veggies (50 calories)

>1 cup green salad (100 calories)

Nighttime:

>5 whole-wheat crackers (100 calories)

>½ tablespoon peanut butter (50 calories)

" I Hate the Way My Boobs Look. "

"Unfortunately, I didn't lose all my baby fat between Ryan and Justin because I was still nursing when I got pregnant. Justin was a bit of a surprise, as we were planning on waiting until Ryan was a year old (I got pregnant when my son Ryan was only nine months old). After Justin was born, I was so busy with the two of them I didn't really have time to worry about losing weight; I just lost it somehow. But running around after them definitely helped! The one body change I see that I was not ready for now that they're both past the one-year mark is the way my boobs look. I'm sure everyone can agree with that, or at least I hope they can! Is there a solution other than a full-out boob job?"

—Elana Cornelius, mother of three-year-old Ryan and two-year-old Justin

Good question, and a very common problem for moms! Because of all the growing and shrinking your breasts do during pregnancy and after, they tend to lose their elasticity and sometimes their shape. And whether or not you decide to breast-feed doesn't really matter because most of the changes occur during pregnancy and after you've given birth. For example, when your milk comes in, your breasts grow. And when you are no longer lactating, they shrink! Simple laws of evolution—or something like that. The point is, you will see some changes in your breasts after having a baby. And whether or not you're comfortable with having a surgical procedure such as a breast lift or breast implants is up to you (I personally am afraid to even get a flu shot so it's pretty safe to say I'm not a good candidate not to mention the fact that implants sag over time).

But is there a natural way to improve the shape and firmness of your breasts? Absolutely! I have two words for you—push-ups. Just like climbing stairs can give you a bubble butt, push-ups can give you the lift you're looking for (see "Coffee Table Workout" in Chapter 9). Push-ups make the muscles that lie beneath your breasts firm and can even pump them up to appear larger. By strengthening the pectoral muscles, you can give a lift to your breasts that will look good on you no matter what size breasts you have. Another exercise that is great for shaping and firming your breasts are dips (see "Coffee Table Workout" in Chapter 9). This exercise also works the pectoral muscles and helps give you the lift and shape you're looking for.

Besides exercises that lift and shape your breasts, there are a few other things you can try. Bust firming creams that contain yeast and other herbal and botanical ingredients are good for firming and toning. It just depends on whether or not you want to spend the money, although they are a lot less expensive than a boob job!

A support bra is always a good choice to help maintain a lift and keep your skin from losing its elasticity. I remember hearing Halle Berry say that she started "sleeping in her bra" when she hit the ripe old age of thirty because gravity had already started working against her. And she hasn't even had a baby!

And last but not least, you can increase your fat intake

and your breasts will get larger but unfortunately it doesn't go just there! Darn! I think it's safe to say that exercise is the best plan for re-shaping and firming your bust line. That, and just being happy with what you have—because it's quality over quantity that matters most.

" Will My Stretch Marks Ever Go Away? "

"I was looking good until the last two weeks of my pregnancy when all of a sudden I got stretch marks! Now my baby is a year old and I'm worried they'll never go away or they'll get darker in the sun. Help!"

Stretch marks are a problem for many women, especially when they go through puberty and toward the end of a pregnancy when the stomach expands the most. Your breasts, thighs, butt, and hips are all susceptible areas for stretch marks, but the good news is they do fade over time. This is when the color usually changes from a red or purplish tone to flesh colored or thin white lines.

In the meantime, one of the best camouflages for stretch marks to help blend them into your skin better is by using self-tanners. Over-the-counter self-tanners can even out pigment and reduce the appearance of stretch marks significantly. But steer away from tanning beds because the skin won't tan evenly and you won't get the same effect. Other creams on the market for stretch marks can be costly and not as effective (although Strivectin and Strixaderm are both used by women on their face to soften the lines around their eyes and is worth a try).

If you do end up having permanent stretch marks, there are treatments at your dermatologist's office that are available, such as micro-dermbrasion and laser treatments. They can be costly and are usually done through several treatments over a period of time but can really help improve the appearance of stretch marks. And if all else fails, do like so many women I know who have stretch marks and do wear a tankini to the beach! No one will ever be the wiser . . .

PAT YOURSELF ON THE BACK

Well, it's time to celebrate. You made it through an entire year and it just keeps getting better and better, doesn't it? Now you can look forward to your baby talking and running and doing so many things that will simply amaze you.

I hope you keep this book around in case you do decide to have another baby one day. And I sincerely hope it helps you remember all the stages you'll go through after giving birth and how a little bit of planning goes a long way. A good friend once reminded me, "It's not the destination that's important; it's the journey." And I find that to be truer today than ever before in my life. Enjoy!

Appendix

SPRI products available at www.spriproducts.com or by calling 1-800-222-7774.

SPRI Jump rope:

Adjustable Plastic Segmented Jump Rope

SPRI Exercise balls:

Professional Plus Xercise Ball—Blue (65cm)

Standard Xercise Ball—White (55cm)

SPRI Resistance Bands:

Resist-a-Band Orange—Very Light

Resist-a-Band Green—Light

Resist-a-Band Blue—medium

Resist-a-Band Purple—heavy

SPRI Weights:

Adjustable Chrome Dumbbell Set—30 Pounds

SPRI Heart Rate Monitor:

Polar Heart Rate Monitor A-5

SPRI Pedometer:

Digital Pedometer

Index

About the Author

LaReine Chabut is a fitness model, actress, writer and mother. The author of *Exercise Balls for Dummies* (Wiley, 2005), she is also a certified fitness instructor and personal trainer. She has served as lead instructor for the workout video series *The Firm* (three million copies sold worldwide) and has graced the covers of such high-profile fitness publications as *Shape, Health, New Body*, and *Runner's World*. LaReine has appeared on national television as a lifestyle and fitness expert teaching women how to get back in shape after having a baby and currently enjoys relationships with Nestlé's Good Start Baby Formula and Nike.

To read more about LaReine Chabut, log on to her website at www.LaReineChabut.com